MW01035825

ISBN: 9781099082849

90-DAY
SMART DIET
1500-CALORIE

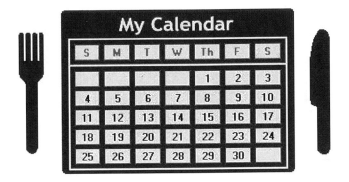

Susan Chen
Gail Johnson, M.S.

NoPaperPress™

NOTE: At publication, the off-the-shelf foods used in portions of this book were widely available in most supermarkets. But food products come and go. So if there is a frozen entrée or soup selection in this diet that is out of stock, or that's been discontinued, or perhaps that you don't like, or that you forgot to pick up while shopping, please substitute another food that has **approximately** the same caloric value and nutritional content. In this regard, many dieters have found the foods listed in the Appendices at the end of this book to be very helpful.

CONTENTS

Day 13 – Pasta with Marinara Sauce (119)
Day 14 - Smoothie (120)
Day 15 – London Broil (121)
Day 16 – Baked Red Snapper (122)
Day 17 – Cajun Chicken Salad (123)
Day 18 – Grilled Swordfish (124)
Day 19 – Chinese Dinner Out (125)
Day 20 – Quick Pasta Puttanesca (126)
Day 21 - Frozen Meat Dinner (127)
Day 22 – Shrimp & Spinach Salad (128)
Day 23 – Beans & Greens Salad (129)
Day 24 – Four Beans Plus Salad (130)
Day 25 – Pan-Broiled Hanger Steak (131)
Day 26 – Grilled Scallops & Polenta (132)
Day 27 – Fettuccine in Summer Sauce (133)
Day 28 – Frozen Chicken Dinner (134)
Day 29 – Barbequed Shrimp & Corn (135)
Day 30 – Cheeseburger Heaven (136)
Day 31 – Baked Sea Bass (137)
Day 32 – Grilled Turkey Tenders (138)
Day 33 – Frozen Fish Dinner (139)
Day 34 – Pasta Rapini (140)
Day 35 – Chicken Dinner Out (141)
Day 36 – Grilled Tilapia (142)
Day 37 – Lo-Cal Beef Stew (143)
Day 38 – Broiled Lamb Chop (144)
Day 39 – Chicken with Veggies (145)
Day 40 – Fish Dinner Out (146)
Day 41 – Pasta e Fagioli (147)
Day 42 – Muffins (148)
Day 43 – Beef Kebob (149)
Day 44 – Baked Haddock (150)
Day 45 – Chicken Cacciatore (151)
Day 46 – Poached Cod (152
Day 47 – Chinese Dinner Out (153)
Day 48 – Healthy Pasta Salad (154)
Day 49 – Frozen Meat Dinner (155)
Day 50 – Pan-Fried Sole (156)
Day 51 – Beans & Greens Salad (157)
Day 52 – Chicken Piccata (158)

Why You Lose Weight

Most experts agree that when the energy value of the food you eat minus waste, equals the sum of your basal metabolic energy plus the energy you expend during physical activity, you will neither gain nor lose weight. They also agree that when you have an energy imbalance, you will either gain or lose weight. In general then:

- **Weight Maintenance** occurs when your food energy intake equals the total energy you expend in daily living. In this case your weight remains stable, i.e., you neither gain nor lose weight.

- **Weight Gain** occurs when your food energy intake is greater than the total energy you expend in daily living. In this case your body stores the extra energy as fat.

- **Weight Loss** occurs when your food energy intake is less than the total energy you expend in daily living. In this case your body converts stored fat (and in some cases muscle) into energy.

The measure of energy, whether in the form of food, physical activity, or heat, is the kilocalorie (hereafter simply called the Calorie). As already mentioned, weight loss occurs when you eat fewer calories than the calories you use in your day-to-day living. This difference in calories is referred to as your calorie deficit. How much weight you lose depends on the magnitude of your calorie deficit. (In technical terms, **the calorie deficit, or calorie difference, is the driving force for weight change**.)

Most people on a weight-loss diet want to know how much weight they will lose – and how fast. Simple metabolic calculations make a rough estimate possible. Physiologists have long known that to lose one pound requires a deficit of approximately 3500 Calories. Therefore, if a person's total calorie deficit over time is known, their weight loss over time can be calculated. (See **"Expected Weight Loss"** - page 8.) **In summary, if you eat and exercise such that you have a calorie deficit you will lose weight!**

The Best Weight Loss Diets

According to the late Dr. Jean Mayer, of Tufts University's Department of Nutrition, a really good weight-loss diet must have the following three characteristics:

1) The diet must provide you with an understanding of weight control as well as the knowledge you need to reduce your weight to the desired level.

2) The diet must help you remain healthy while you are losing weight.

3) The diet must lead you to a healthier way of eating and exercising that will, in the long term, help you keep off the weight you have lost.

Why the 90-Day Smart Diet?

Experts agree that a diet that promotes weight loss over a relatively longer time period is healthier and the weight loss is likely to be more permanent. These experts recommend you choose a nutritious diet that results in a weight loss of approximately 2 pounds per week – which amounts to about 26 lbs in 90 days. The *90-Day Smart Diet* fits the bill!

Expected Weight Loss

On the *90-Day Smart Diet - 1500 Calorie Edition*, **most women lose 18 to 28 pounds.** Smaller women, older women and less active women lose a bit less and larger women, younger women and more active women often lose much more.

On the *90-Day Smart Diet - 1500 Calorie Edition*, **most men lose 28 to 38 pounds**. Smaller men, older men and less active men will lose a tad less and larger men, younger men and more active men frequently lose much more.

Exactly how much weight you will lose depends on how much you weigh, your age and your activity level. For the full story see *Weight Control - U.S. Edition* by Vincent W. Antonetti, Ph.D., an eBook also published by NoPaperPress.

Smart Diet Info

The *90-Day Smart Diet* contains meal plans, recipes and guidance for 90 fat-melting days! How long you stay on the diet, 10 days, 45 days, or all 90 days – depends on how much weight you want to lose.

The Daily Menu for **Day 1** is on page 16. Associated with each of the 90 days is a "**Recipe of the Day**" starting on page 107 with a "Diet Tip of the Day."

Even though the *90-Day Smart Diet* adheres to the United States Department of Agriculture balanced diet recommendations, the *90-Day Smart Diet* may not be appropriate for everyone, such as individuals with illnesses such as heart disease, diabetes, food allergies, etc. Make sure you check with your physician before starting this diet, or any diet.

First a Medical Exam

Everyone should at the very least have a medical assessment, or exam, before starting a weight loss diet. Why? You need to make sure your health will allow you to lower your caloric intake and increase your physical activity. Depending on your age and state of health, the medical checkup may be as simple as a visit to a physician who is familiar with your medical history, or it may be a thorough physical exam. The physician conducting the medical exam should be made aware of and should approve the specific weight loss diet you're planning. Additionally, if you are going to engage in some sort of physical activity in conjunction with this diet and especially if you have been totally inactive, or if you have or suspect you have cardiovascular disease or other health problems, or if you are obese, or if you are 40 or older, before embarking on the physical fitness portion of your weight control program you should have a stress test supervised by a physician. Finally, your physician can tell you how much and what type of exercise is right for you, how much you should weigh, and prescribe a realistic weight- loss goal.

Eat Smart

No single food can supply all the nutrients you need in the amounts you need. The most important factors in nutrition are variety, variety, variety! **Variety is the key to a nutritious diet.** As a means of setting strategies for food selection, the U.S. Department of Health and Human Services and the Department of Agriculture issue Dietary Guidelines every five years. The latest Dietary Guidelines describe a healthy diet as one that:
- Emphasizes fruits, vegetables, whole grains, and fat-free or low-fat milk products.
- Includes fish, poultry, lean meats, beans and nuts.
- Is low in saturated fats, trans fats, cholesterol, salt (sodium) and added sugars.
The latest guidelines encourage adults to consume a variety of nutrient-dense foods and beverages within their caloric needs. The afore mentioned U.S. government agencies recommend how much should be eaten from each of the basic food groups (i.e., from the fruit group, vegetable group, grains group, meat and beans group, dairy group, and oils group) to meet your caloric goal – whether you are trying to lose weight or maintain weight. All this information and more can be found in *Eat Smart - U.S. Edition* an eBook published by NoPaperPress.

Even though most adults can get all the vitamins and minerals they need by merely consuming a variety of nutritious foods (from the fruit group, the vegetable group, the grains group, the meat and beans group, the milk group, and the oils group), many physicians recommend a daily multi-vitamin/mineral supplement – just in case you don't eat the way you should.

9

Be aware that some micronutrients, such as the fat-soluble vitamin A, can be harmful if taken in large quantities. To be safe your multi-vitamin/mineral supplement should contain no more than 100 percent of the recommended dietary allowance (RDA) for each vitamin or mineral. Generally, you don't need the high doses in multi-vitamin/mineral supplements labeled "therapeutic" or "extra-strength." There may be medical reasons for taking larger amounts of a vitamin or mineral than the RDA provides, but check with your doctor first.

Tossed Salad

One of the dinner mainstays in the *90-Day Smart Diet* is a "Tossed Salad." To prepare your "Tossed Salad" start with a bowl that has a volume of at least 16 ounces, or 2 cups. First add about 1 cup of either green leaf lettuce, Romaine lettuce or a Mesclun mix. Then add at least a half cup of other veggies such as broccoli, celery, cucumber, spinach, or watercress. This vegetable combination will, on average, total about 35 Calories.

You'll be eating a "Tossed Salad" just about every day at dinnertime. Remember that variety is the key to a nutritious diet. So be sure to vary the ingredients of the salad. Top your Tossed Salad with 1½ tablespoons of any light salad dressing available at your local supermarket that contains no more than 25 Calories per tablespoon. Some of our favorites are:

- **Ken's Steakhouse Fat Free Raspberry Pecan**
- **Kraft Light Done Right House Italian**
- **Newman's Lighten Up! Balsamic Vinaigrette**
- **Wishbone Just 2 Good Honey Dijon**

Your "Tossed Salad" with salad dressing will cost you roughly 70 Calories but will be packed with lots of health-giving vitamins, minerals and fiber.

About Bread

First understand that bread, more specifically whole-grain breads, are good sources of complex carbohydrates and dietary fiber, as well as the B vitamins (thiamin, riboflavin, niacin, and folate), vitamin E, and minerals (iron, magnesium and selenium). In recent years, however, sliced bread loaves have gotten larger, as have the bread slices inside these loaves. Just a few years ago the standard slice of bread contained about 65 to 70 Calories – now most are 100 plus Calories.

The 90-*Day Smart Diet* requires whole-grain bread at 70 Calories per slice. Quite a few bakers sell thin sliced or "light" sliced bread. The difficult part is finding a whole grain thin sliced or "light" bread (with about 70 Calories per slice). Whatever the brand, make sure the first word in the Ingredients list is "whole." "Pepperidge Farm Small Slice 100% Whole Wheat" is a good choice. It's whole grain, has 70 Calories per slice and it tastes good too.

Substituting Foods

If there is a food listed in the **90-Day Smart Diet** that you don't like, or perhaps that you forgot to pick up while shopping, you probably can exchange or substitute another food in its place – a technique used by dieticians. Exchanging a food listed in a diet for another food with approximately equal caloric value and nutritional content is the foundation of many successful long-term diets. Substitution possibilities are almost endless but have to be done carefully. The easiest substitutions are those within the same food group, such as exchanging one vegetable variety for another, or a glass of milk for a cup of yogurt. More sophisticated exchanges cross food groups, such as replacing 3½ ounces of turkey with a tablespoon of peanut butter on a piece of whole-wheat bread. Both foods are complete protein and both contain about 175 Calories. (Refer to a good online calorie table.) With some understanding and experience, you can use a calorie table to help you substitute foods called for in the **90-Day Smart Diet** with equal calorie foods from the same food group.

Breakfast: You may substitute any cereal for any other wholesome cereal. For example, if you're not crazy about having Shredded Wheat for breakfast on Day 6, substitute Wheat Chex or Cheerios, etc. But remember to adjust the amount of cereal to account for the calorie difference between brands. If you don't like the soft-boiled egg called for on Day 9, cook a fried egg instead. And if Cantaloupe is on the menu but is not in season, replace cantaloupe with a half cup of orange juice – both contain about 50 Calories.

Snacks: Again, where 6 ounces of yogurt is specified you may substitute an 8-ounce glass of skim milk, but to maintain a nutritionally balanced diet keep this snack a dairy selection. Similarly, when fruit is on the agenda, you may select any type of fruit but do not stray from the fruit group. Nuts and popcorn can be interchanged at will. Specified convenient brand-name snacks, such as Skinny Cow ice cream, Kashi Granola bars, Nabisco 100 Calorie Pack cookies and Orville Redenbacher's Smart Pop Popcorn should be widely available but other equivalent brands may be substituted if need be. Just make sure the substitute snack has the same calorie count, or very close, to the specified snack.

Two Nights – No Cooking

Everyone deserves a break from the grind of preparing dinner after coming home from work. So the **90-Day Smart Diet** gives you two days off per week! Notice that one night a week the meal plan calls for a frozen dinner and on a second night during the week you're encouraged to eat out. There are, however, some rules and caveats involved – these are covered in the next two sections.

Frozen Dinner Rules

In general, a frozen dinner should not be a meal in itself. Make sure you add a salad, fruit, bread etc. The frozen dinner you choose should come with at least one cup of cooked vegetables. If your frozen dinner doesn't measure up, add your own frozen, fresh or canned vegetables. And look for dinners with no more than 800 mg of sodium. In addition, make sure the dinner you choose has no more than 30 percent of the daily value for total fat. Appendix A on page 196 contains a comprehensive tabulation of reasonably good frozen dinner choices. And on the days when a frozen dinner is specified, you will be given a calorie goal for the frozen dinner. For example, Day 5 calls for frozen fish dinner with a maximum allowable 340 Calories. If you choose a frozen fish dinner that contains less than 340 Calories, you may spend the unused calories any way you wish.

Moreover, on those nights when you just don't have the energy or time to cook, you can always substitute a frozen dinner for the "Recipe of the Day" or the entree listed in the meal plan. For example, Day 2 calls for Herb-Crusted Cod for dinner. The total calorie count for dinner is 520. In place of the cod, any combination of a frozen fish dinner and side dishes (salads, etc) with a total calorie content close to 520 would be an acceptable, albeit not as tasty, alternative.

Eating Out Challenges

You may eat out once a week. When you're on a diet, however, eating in a restaurant can be a challenge, because most restaurant portions are huge, and can easily total more than 1000 Calories. On the **90-Day Smart Diet**, a dinner type (i.e., fish, chicken, etc) and a calorie target is specified. For example Day 7 of the 1500 Calorie diet calls for a chicken dinner and allows you 630 Calories.

First, you need to choose a restaurant where you have a fighting chance to achieve your calorie goal. Next, order something simple, such as broiled fish with steamed vegetables and brown rice. Tell the waiter you want no sauce, no gravy, nothing added. Then, knowing your calorie objective, and that most fish and chicken are about 50 Calories per ounce, most steamed vegetable servings average approximately 50 Calories per cup, and rice is about 100 Calories per ½ cup, decide how much to eat – and take the remainder home. If fresh fruit is not an option, pass on dessert and have the evening snack specified in the 90-Day Smart Diet meal plan for that day.

Smart Diet Notes

1) Coffee or tea may be caffeinated or decaf. If desired, skim milk and a sugar substitute may be added to coffee or tea. And **Soy or Almond** milk may be used instead of skim milk.

2) Fried eggs or scrambled eggs should be cooked in a pan coated with a non-stick cooking spray. Hard-boiled eggs may be substituted for fried, scrambled or soft-boiled eggs.

3) Cereals should be whole grain and unsweetened. At the top of the list are Old-fashioned Oatmeal, Wheatena and Shredded Wheat. Among other reasonably healthy choices are Cheerios, Wheat Chex, Wheaties, some Kashi cereals and Farina. When blueberries are in season, you may **substitute blueberries for raisins** added to your cereal. (Approx. substitution ratio = 2 blueberries for one raisin.)

4) Bread may be either plain or toasted whole grain, such as whole wheat, whole rye or pumpernickel. Look for whole grain varieties that contain 70 Calories per slice. If desired, bread may be sprayed with a zero-calorie butter substitute.

5) When soup in a microwaveable bowl is specified, eat only one serving (8 ounces) unless otherwise noted. (Microwaveable bowls usually contain about two servings.)

6) Use freely as desired: clear unsweetened coffee, clear unsweetened tea, water, seltzer water and any diet soda, clear soups without fat, bouillon, and seasonings such as mustard, cinnamon, dill, herbs, red and black pepper, curry, vinegar, lemon juice and sections, and dill and sour pickles.

7) Use only lean cuts of meat trimmed of all visible fat. Poultry should be limited to chicken or turkey breasts (white meat only and skinless).

8) When canned tuna or salmon is specified, use fish **packed in water**.

9) When the diet calls for turkey bacon, make sure the brand you buy has no more than 35 Calories per slice.

10) An unlimited amount of green salad may be eaten, but the salad dressing should be as specified.

11) If it's more convenient, any food item may be moved to any part of the day and combined with any meal or snack.

12) If you cannot find the exact item called for in the diet (because it's out of stock or discontinued), substitute a comparable food (of the same type and close caloric value).

13) Take a daily **multi-vitamin/mineral supplement**. This is important when you're on a diet – as a kind of insurance policy.

Keeping It Off

Within five years, more than 90 percent of all dieters regain every pound they have lost. Why? In most cases it's because after losing weight most people eventually revert to their pre-diet eating and exercising habits, and this inevitably leads to their regaining the weight they lost – and often more. Obviously after a diet you weigh less. The fact is the less you weigh, the less you need to eat to sustain your lower weight.

A study, published in the *Annals of Internal Medicine*, that followed 4,000 people for three decades suggests that in the long term, 90 percent of men and 70 percent of women will become overweight. Interestingly, half of the men and women in the study, who had made it well into adulthood without a weight problem, ultimately also became overweight and a third actually became obese. The point being that you can never become complacent. You must continually watch your weight because we are all at risk of becoming overweight.

The key to long-term weight control success is knowledge and understanding, combined of course with desire and self-discipline. Once you reach your weight goal, I suggest you read ***Weight Maintenance - U.S. Edition*** by Vincent Antonetti, Ph.D. (also published by NoPaperPress) – absolutely the best weight maintenance book, or eBook, on the market.

1500 CALORIE DAILY MENUS

Day 1 1500 Calorie Meal Plan

BREAKFAST	Calories	Totals
Grapefruit (½)	75	
Scrambled egg (See Notes - page 13)	80	
Turkey Bacon (2 slices)	70	
Whole-grain toast (1 slice) (See page 10)	70	
Coffee (Page 13)	10	305 Cal
SNACK		
Yogurt (6 oz nonfat, any flavor)*	90	
Coffee or tea	10	100 Cal
* Such as Dannon Lite & Fit. (Buy 32 oz & use 6 oz.)		
LUNCH		
Ham (2 oz) with mustard on 2 slices rye bread	290	
Pickle spear	0	
Small bunch of grapes	65	
Hot or iced tea	10	365 Cal
SNACK		
Fresh fruit in season (apple, peach, etc)	70	
Coffee or tea	10	80 Cal
DINNER		
Chicken w Peppers & Onions (Day 1 Recipe page 107)	250	
Sautéed red peppers with onions (Day 1 recipe)	70	
Green beans - steamed, & mashed cauliflower	55	
Large tossed salad with 1½ Tbsp low-cal dressing	70	
Whole-grain bread (1 slice)	70	
Water with lemon wedge	10	525 Cal
SNACK		
Popcorn Mini Bag**	110	
Coffee or tea	10	120 Cal
** Such as Orville Redenbacher's Smart Pop.		1495 Cal

16

Day 2 1500 Calorie Meal Plan

BREAKFAST	Calories	Totals
Orange juice (½ cup)	50	
Wheaties (¾ cup) + ½ cup skim milk + ½ banana	190	
Whole-grain toast (1 slice)	70	
Coffee	10	320 Cal
SNACK		
Fresh fruit in season (apple, pear, etc)	70	
Coffee or tea	10	80 Cal
LUNCH		
Soup (Appendix B - page 202)	110	
Turkey breast (2 oz) on 2 slices rye bread	210	
Pickle spear	0	
Lettuce & tomato slices	20	
Hot or iced tea	10	350 Cal
SNACK		
Popcorn Mini Bag	110	
Coffee or tea	10	120 Cal
DINNER		
Baked Herb-Crusted Cod (Day 2 Recipe page 108)	230	
Spinach (½ cup) steamed with garlic & drizzled	100	
Asparagus (7 spear cooked & drained)	20	
Baked potato (medium size) (No Butter!)	100	
Gelatin dessert (unsweetened)	10	
Water with lemon wedge	10	470 Cal
SNACK		
Skinny Cow Ice Cream Sandwich	140	
Coffee or tea	10	150 Cal
		1490 Cal

17

Day 3 1500 Calorie Meal Plan

BREAKFAST	Calories	Totals
Fresh or frozen strawberries (½ cup)	25	
French toasted English Muffin (Day 3 Recipe page 109)	270	
Light syrup (1 Tbsp)	30	
Coffee	10	335 Cal
SNACK		
Yogurt (6 oz – nonfat, any flavor)	90	
Coffee or tea	10	100 Cal
LUNCH		
Salad (3 oz canned tuna, 1 tsp Evoo, onions, celery)	175	
Lettuce & tomato wedges	20	
Rye bread (1 slice)	70	
Fresh fruit in season (apple, peach, etc)	70	
Coffee or tea	10	345 Cal
SNACK		
Handful unsalted mixed nuts	100	
Coffee or tea	10	110 Cal
DINNER		
Broiled veal chop (4 oz lean)	200	
Corn on the cob (1 medium ear) (No Butter!)	100	
Broccoli (½ cup steamed & drizzled with 1 tsp	70	
Large tossed salad with 1½ Tbsp low-cal dressing	70	
Water with lemon wedge	10	450 Cal
SNACK		
Skinny Cow Ice Cream Sandwich	140	
Coffee or tea	10	150 Cal
		1490 Cal

Day 4 1500 Calorie Meal Plan

BREAKFAST	Calories	Totals
Grapefruit (½)	75	
Cheerios (1 cup) + ½ cup skim milk + about 15 raisins*	190	
Coffee	10	275 Cal
SNACK		
Fresh fruit in season (apple, plum, etc)	70	
Coffee or tea	10	80 Cal
LUNCH		
Cottage cheese (1 cup low fat)	180	
Large tossed salad with 2 Tbsp low-cal dressing	85	
Small whole-grain roll	80	
Hot or iced tea	10	355 Cal
SNACK		
Handful unsalted mixed nuts	100	
Coffee or tea	10	110 Cal
DINNER		
Meat Loaf (Day 4 Recipe - page 110)	290	
One-half acorn squash (baked with ½ tsp maple	90	
Spinach (½ cup steamed & drizzled with 1 tsp	70	
Romaine lettuce, tomato slices & 1 Tbsp low-cal	45	
Gelatin dessert (unsweetened)	10	
Water with lemon wedge	10	515 Cal
SNACK		
Two small cookies (sugar, choc chip, …- check calories!)	160	
Coffee or tea	10	170 Cal
* See Notes page 13 re substituting blueberries for raisins.		1505 Cal

Day 5 1500 Calorie Meal Plan

BREAKFAST	Calories	Totals
Cantaloupe (½ medium)	50	
Fried egg	80	
Toasted raisin bread (1 slice)	75	
Coffee	10	215 Cal
SNACK		
Yogurt (6 oz nonfat, any flavor)	90	
Coffee or tea	10	100 Cal
LUNCH		
Subway 6" (Ham, Cheese + veggies)*	260	
Canned pineapple (1 cup, no-sugar-added juice)	80	
Water with lemon wedge	10	350 Cal
* On 6" half wheat roll.		
SNACK		
Dark chocolate (1 oz)	150	
Coffee or tea	10	160 Cal
DINNER		
Frozen fish dinner (Day 5 Recipe - page 111)	340	
Large tossed salad with 1½ Tbsp low-cal dressing	70	
Whole-grain bread (1 slice)	70	
Fresh fruit in season (apple, peach, etc)	70	
Water with lemon wedge	10	560 Cal
SNACK		
Popcorn Mini Bag	110	
Coffee or tea	10	120 Cal
		1505 Cal

Day 6 1500 Calorie Meal Plan

BREAKFAST	Calories	Totals
Tomato juice (½ cup)	20	
Shredded Wheat (1 cup) + ½ cup skim milk + ½	265	
Coffee	10	295 Cal
SNACK		
Handful unsalted mixed nuts	100	
Coffee or tea	10	110 Cal
LUNCH		
Leftover meat loaf (½ of Day 4 serving) w ketchup	155	
Small whole-grain roll	80	
Lettuce	0	
Fresh or frozen berries (½ cup)	50	
Hot or iced tea	10	295 Cal
SNACK		
Yogurt (6 oz, nonfat, any flavor)	90	
Coffee or tea	10	100 Cal
DINNER		
Pizza (Day 6 Recipe - page 112)	350	
Large tossed salad with 1½ Tbsp low-cal dressing	70	
Fresh fruit in season (apple, peach, etc)	70	
Glass of red wine (4 oz)	100	
Water with lemon wedge	10	600 Cal
SNACK		
100-Calorie Pack Cookies*	100	
Coffee or tea	10	110 Cal
* For example, Nabisco Oreo/Chips Ahoy/etc		1510 Cal

Day 7 1500 Calorie Meal Plan

BREAKFAST	Calories	Totals
Cantaloupe (½ medium)	50	
Oatmeal (½ cup dry) + ½ cup skim milk + 15 raisins	220	
Coffee	10	280 Cal
SNACK		
Fresh fruit in season (apple, plum, etc)	70	
Coffee or tea	10	80 Cal
LUNCH		
Chorizo, Egg & Cheese*	260	
Small bunch of grapes	50	
Hot or iced tea	10	320 Cal
* Hot Pockets (wrap) or if unavailable an equivalent food.		
SNACK		
Handful unsalted mixed nuts	100	
Coffee or tea	10	110 Cal
DINNER		
Eat Out – Chicken dinner (Day 7 Recipe - page 113)		
Max allowable calories	630	630 Cal
SNACK		
Graham crackers (2 squares)	60	
Coffee or tea	10	70 Cal
		1490 Cal

Day 8 1500 Calorie Meal Plan

BREAKFAST	Calories	Totals
Cantaloupe (½ medium)	50	
Wheaties (¾ cup) + ½ cup skim milk + ½ banana	190	
Whole grain toast (1 slice)	70	
Coffee	10	320 Cal
SNACK		
Handful unsalted mixed nuts	100	
Coffee or tea	10	110 Cal
LUNCH		
Roast beef (2 oz) sandwich on whole-grain bread	305	
Lettuce & tomato slices	20	
Hot or ice tea	10	335 Cal
SNACK		
Popcorn Mini Bag	110	
Coffee or tea	10	120 Cal
DINNER		
Baked salmon with salsa (Day 8 Recipe - page 114)	215	
Baked summer squash and zucchini	40	
Medium tomato - sliced	20	
Brown rice (½ cup – after cooking)	100	
Large tossed salad with 1½ Tbsp low-cal dressing	70	
Water	0	445 Cal
SNACK		
Graham crackers (4 squares)	120	
Skim milk (4 oz)	45	165 Cal
		1495 Cal

Day 9 1500 Calorie Meal Plan

BREAKFAST	Calories	Totals
Orange juice (½ cup)	50	
Soft-boiled egg	80	
Whole-grain toast (2 slices)	140	
Coffee	10	280 Cal
SNACK		
Yogurt (6 oz, nonfat, any flavor)	90	
Coffee or tea	10	100 Cal
LUNCH		
Salad (3 oz canned tuna, 1 tsp Evoo, onions, celery)	175	
Lettuce & tomato wedges + rye bread (1 slice)	90	
Fresh fruit in season – (apple, pear, etc)	70	
Coffee or tea	10	345 Cal
SNACK		
Handful unsalted mixed nuts	100	
Coffee or tea	10	110 Cal
DINNER		
Veggie burger – (1 patty) (Day 9 Recipe - page 115)	100	
Low-fat cheddar cheese (1 thin slice)	50	
Seeded hamburger roll	140	
Beets (3 small, boiled, skinned & sliced)	45	
Large tossed salad with 1½ Tbsp low-cal dressing	70	
Fresh fruit in season (apple, peach, etc)	70	
Water with lemon wedge	10	485 Cal
SNACK		
Graham crackers (4 squares)	120	
Skim milk (6 oz)	65	185 Cal
		1505 Cal

Day 10 1500 Calorie Meal Plan

BREAKFAST	Calories	Totals
Orange juice (½ cup)	50	
Wild blueberry pancakes (Day 10 Recipe - page 116)	190	
Turkey bacon (2 slices)	70	
Light syrup (1½ Tbsp)	45	
Coffee	10	365 Cal
SNACK		
Yogurt (6 oz, nonfat, any flavor)	90	
Coffee or tea	10	100 Cal
LUNCH		
Peanut butter (2 Tbsp) on 2 slices bread	340	
Skim milk (6 oz)	65	
Water with lemon wedge	10	415 Cal
SNACK		
Fresh fruit in season – (apple, pear, etc)	70	
Coffee or tea	10	80 Cal
DINNER		
Broiled pork chop (about 4 oz of meat - trimmed of fat)	260	
Green peas (½ cup)	55	
Tomato & cucumber salad with 1½ Tbsp low-cal	70	
Water with lemon wedge	10	395 Cal
SNACK		
Skinny Cow Ice Cream Sandwich	140	
Coffee or tea	10	150 Cal
		1505 Cal

Day 11 1500 Calorie Meal Plan

BREAKFAST	Calories	Totals
Fresh sliced orange	75	
Cheerios (1 cup) + ½ cup skim milk + about 15 raisins	190	
Whole-grain toast (1 slice)	70	
Coffee	10	345 Cal
SNACK		
Handful unsalted mixed nuts	100	
Coffee or tea	10	110 Cal
LUNCH		
Chicken, Bacon Ranch*	270	
Fresh fruit in season (apple, peach, etc)	70	
Diet soda or water	0	340 Cal
* Hot Pockets (wrap) or if unavailable an equivalent food.		
SNACK		
Fresh fruit in season (peach, plum, etc)	70	
Coffee or tea	10	80 Cal
DINNER		
Grilled chicken sausage (2 links about 2½ oz per link)	180	
Artichoke-bean salad (Day 11 Recipe - page 117)	190	
Green beans (¼ lb – steamed)	25	
Whole-grain bread (1 slice)	70	
Water with lemon wedge	10	475 Cal
SNACK		
Skinny Cow Ice Cream Sandwich	140	
Coffee or tea	10	150 Cal
		1500 Cal

Day 12 1500 Calorie Meal Plan

BREAKFAST	Calories	Totals
Grapefruit (½)	75	
Scrambled egg	80	
Turkey bacon (2 slices)	70	
Whole-grain toast (1 slice)	70	
Coffee	10	305 Cal
SNACK		
Yogurt (6 oz, nonfat, any flavor)	90	
Coffee or tea	10	100 Cal
LUNCH		
Soup (Appendix B - page 202)	150	
Tomato slices with ¼ cup chopped fresh basil + 1	60	
Whole-grain bread (1 slice)	70	
Hot or iced tea	10	280 Cal
SNACK		
Fresh fruit in season (peach, plum, etc)	70	
Coffee or tea	10	80 Cal
DINNER		
Eat Out – Fish dinner (Day 12 Recipe - page 118)		
Max allowable calories	595	595 Cal
SNACK		
Graham crackers (4 squares)	120	
Coffee or tea	10	130 Cal
		1500 Cal

Day 13 1500 Calorie Meal Plan

BREAKFAST	Calories	Totals
Orange juice (½ cup)	50	
Shredded Wheat (1 cup) + ½ cup skim milk + ½ banana	260	
Coffee	10	320 Cal
SNACK		
Handful unsalted mixed nuts	100	
Coffee or tea	10	110 Cal
LUNCH		
Turkey frank (2 oz) with mustard & relish	150	
Hot-dog bun	130	
Hot or iced tea	10	290 Cal
SNACK		
Kashi TLC Chewy Granola Bar	140	
Coffee or tea	10	150 Cal
DINNER		
Pasta with Marinara sauce (Day 13 Recipe - page 119)	225	
Large tossed salad with 1½ Tbsp low-cal dressing	70	
Fresh fruit in season (peach, plum, etc)	70	
Glass of red wine (4 oz)	100	
Water with lemon wedge	10	475 Cal
SNACK		
Skinny Cow Ice Cream Sandwich	140	
Coffee or tea	10	150 Cal
		1495 Cal

Day 14 1500 Calorie Meal Plan

BREAKFAST	Calories	Totals
Cantaloupe (½ medium)	50	
Low-Cal Smoothie (Day 14 Recipe - page 120)	220	
Coffee	10	280 Cal
SNACK		
Handful unsalted mixed nuts	100	
Coffee or tea	10	110 Cal
LUNCH		
Grilled Swiss cheese sandwich (2 oz low-fat cheese)	320	
Pickle spear	0	
Hot or iced tea	10	330 Cal
SNACK		
100-Calorie Pack Cookies	100	
Coffee or tea	10	110 Cal
DINNER		
Frozen chicken dinner (Day 28 Recipe - page 134)	300	
Large tossed salad with 1½ Tbsp low-cal dressing	70	
Whole-grain bread (1 slice)	70	
Fresh fruit in season (apple, peach, etc)	70	
Water with lemon wedge	10	520 Cal
SNACK		
Dark chocolate (1 oz)	150	
Coffee or tea	10	160 Cal
		1510 Cal

Day 15 1500 Calorie Meal Plan

BREAKFAST	Calories	Totals
Fresh or frozen strawberries (1 cup)	50	
French toasted English Muffin (Day 3 Recipe page 109)	270	
Light syrup (1 Tbsp)	30	
Coffee	10	360 Cal
SNACK		
Yogurt (6 oz, nonfat, any flavor)	90	
Coffee or tea	10	100 Cal
LUNCH		
Salad (3 oz canned tuna, 1 tsp Evoo, onions, celery)	175	
Lettuce & tomato wedges	20	
Rye bread (1 slice)	70	
Coffee or tea	10	275 Cal
SNACK		
Handful unsalted mixed nuts	100	
Coffee or tea	10	110 Cal
DINNER		
London broil (Day 15 Recipe - page 121)	320	
Brown rice (½ cup – after cooking)	100	
Steamed broccoli (1 cup – after cooking)	50	
Fresh fruit in season (apple, plum, etc)	70	
Water with lemon wedge	10	550 Cal
SNACK		
100-Calorie Pack Cookies	100	
Coffee or tea	10	110 Cal
		1505 Cal

Day 16 1500 Calorie Meal Plan

BREAKFAST	Calories	Totals
Orange juice (½ cup)	50	
Kashi GoLean (1 cup) + ½ cup skim milk + ½ banana	235	
Coffee	10	295 Cal
SNACK		
Fresh fruit in season (peach, plum, etc)	70	
Coffee or tea	10	80 Cal
LUNCH		
Soup (Appendix B - page 202)	120	
Small whole-grain roll	80	
Lettuce and sliced tomato with 1 Tbsp low-cal	45	
Unsweetened apple sauce (½ cup)	45	
Hot or iced tea	10	300 Cal
SNACK		
Two small cookies	160	
Coffee or tea	10	170 Cal
DINNER		
Baked red snapper (Day 16 Recipe - page 122)	215	
Wild rice mix (Day 16 Recipe)	160	
Green beans & tomato	75	
Yogurt (6 oz, nonfat, any flavor)	90	
Water	0	540 Cal
SNACK		
Popcorn Mini Bag	110	
Coffee or tea	10	120 Cal
		1505 Cal

Day 17 1500 Calorie Meal Plan

BREAKFAST	Calories	Totals
Cantaloupe (½ medium)	50	
Fried egg	80	
Turkey bacon (2 slices)	70	
Toasted raisin bread (1 slice)	75	
Coffee	10	285 Cal
SNACK		
Yogurt (6 oz, nonfat, any flavor)	90	
Coffee or tea	10	100 Cal
LUNCH		
Ham & White Cheddar*	270	
Banana (medium)	100	
Coffee or tea	0	370 Cal
* Hot Pockets (wrap) or if unavailable an equivalent food.		
SNACK		
Handful unsalted mixed nuts	100	
Coffee or tea	10	110 Cal
DINNER		
Cajun chicken salad (Day 17 Recipe - page 123)	330	
Whole-grain bread (1 slice)	70	
Fresh fruit in season (apple, plum, etc)	70	
Water	0	470 Cal
SNACK		
Dark chocolate (1 oz)	150	
Coffee or tea	10	160 Cal
		1500 Cal

32

Day 18 1500 Calorie Meal Plan

BREAKFAST	Calories	Totals
Grapefruit (½)	75	
Cheerios (1 cup) + ½ cup skim milk + about 15 raisins	190	
Coffee	10	275 Cal
SNACK		
Handful unsalted mixed nuts	100	
Coffee or tea	10	110 Cal
LUNCH		
Subway 6" (Roast Beef, Cheese + veggies)*	245	
Large tossed salad with 1½ Tbsp low-cal dressing	70	
Hot or iced tea	10	325 Cal
* On 6" half wheat roll.		
SNACK		
Fresh fruit in season (peach, plum, etc)	70	
Coffee or tea	10	80 Cal
DINNER		
Grilled swordfish (Day 18 Recipe - page 124)	250	
Grilled potatoes (Day 18 Recipe)	100	
Grilled cherry tomatoes (Day 18 Recipe)	45	
Spinach ½ cup steamed with garlic & drizzled with Evoo	50	
Whole-grain bread (1 slice)	70	
Water with lemon wedge	10	525 Cal
SNACK		
Two small cookies	160	
Coffee or tea	10	170 Cal
		1485 Cal

Day 19 1500 Calorie Meal Plan

BREAKFAST	Calories	Totals
Grapefruit (½)	75	
Scrambled egg	80	
Whole-grain toast (1 slice)	70	
Coffee	10	235 Cal
SNACK		
Yogurt (6 oz, nonfat, any flavor)	90	
Coffee or tea	10	100 Cal
LUNCH		
Soup (Appendix B - page 202)	100	
Turkey (1 oz) on 1 slice of rye bread (½ sandwich)	120	
Lettuce & tomato slices	20	
Hot or iced tea	10	250 Cal
SNACK		
Fresh fruit in season (peach, plum, etc)	70	
Coffee or tea	10	80 Cal
DINNER		
Eat Out – Chinese food (Day 19 Recipe - page 125)		
Max allowable calories	640	640 Cal
SNACK		
Graham crackers (4 squares)	120	
Skim milk (6 oz)	70	190 Cal
		1495 Cal

34

Day 20 1500 Calorie Meal Plan

BREAKFAST	Calories	Totals
Tomato juice (½ cup)	20	
Shredded Wheat (1 cup) + ½ cup skim milk + ½ banana	260	
Coffee	10	290 Cal
SNACK		
Handful unsalted mixed nuts	100	
Coffee or tea	10	110 Cal
LUNCH		
Ham (2 oz) with mustard on 2 slices rye bread	290	
Pickle spear	0	
Hot or iced tea	10	300 Cal
SNACK		
Yogurt (6 oz, nonfat, any flavor)	90	
Coffee or tea	10	100 Cal
DINNER		
Spaghetti alla Puttanesca (Day 20 Recipe - page 126)	345	
Large tossed salad with 1½ Tbsp low-cal dressing	70	
Italian or French bread (1 slice)	80	
Glass of red wine (4 oz)	100	
Water	0	595 Cal
SNACK		
100-Calorie Pack Cookies	100	
Coffee or tea	10	110 Cal
		1505 Cal

Day 21 1500 Calorie Meal Plan

BREAKFAST	Calories	Totals
Cantaloupe (½ medium)	50	
Oatmeal (½ cup dry) + ½ cup skim milk + 15 raisins	220	
Whole-grain toast (1 slice)	70	
Coffee	10	350 Cal
SNACK		
Handful unsalted mixed nuts	100	
Coffee or tea	10	110 Cal
LUNCH		
Turkey breast (2 oz) on 2 slices whole-grain bread	245	
Lettuce, tomato and Tbsp light mayo	35	
Pickle spear	0	
Fresh fruit in season (peach, plum, etc)	70	
Water	0	350 Cal
SNACK		
Yogurt (6 oz, nonfat, any flavor)	90	
Coffee or tea	10	100 Cal
DINNER		
Frozen meat dinner (Day 21 Recipe - page 127)	300	
Large tossed salad with 1½ Tbsp low-cal dressing	70	
Whole-grain bread (1 slice)	70	
Water	0	440 Cal
SNACK		
Dark chocolate (1 oz)	150	
Coffee or tea	10	160 Cal
		1510 Cal

36

Day 22 1500 Calorie Meal Plan

BREAKFAST	Calories	Totals
Fresh or frozen strawberries (1 cup)	25	
French toasted English Muffin (Day 3 Recipe - page 109)	270	
Light syrup (1½ Tbsp)	45	
Coffee	10	350 Cal
SNACK		
Yogurt (6 oz, nonfat, any flavor)	90	
Coffee or tea	10	100 Cal
LUNCH		
Southwest-Style Taco*	270	
Small bunch of grapes	50	
Diet soda or water	0	320 Cal
* Hot Pockets (wrap)		
SNACK		
Popcorn Mini Bag	110	
Coffee or tea	10	120 Cal
DINNER		
Shrimp & spinach salad (Day 22 Recipe - page 128)	310	
Whole-grain bread (1 slice)	70	
Fresh fruit in season (apple, peach, etc)	70	
Water	0	450 Cal
SNACK		
Skinny Cow Ice Cream Sandwich	140	
Coffee or tea	10	150 Cal
		1490 Cal

37

Day 23 1500 Calorie Meal Plan

BREAKFAST	Calories	Totals
Cantaloupe (½ medium)	50	
Wheaties (¾ cup) + ½ cup skim milk + ½ banana	190	
Whole-grain toast (1 slice)	70	
Coffee	10	320 Cal
SNACK		
Handful unsalted mixed nuts	100	
Coffee or tea	10	110 Cal
LUNCH		
Ham (2 oz) with mustard on 2 slices rye bread	300	
Pickle spear	0	
Hot or iced tea	10	310 Cal
SNACK		
Yogurt (6 oz, nonfat, any flavor)	90	
Coffee or tea	10	100 Cal
DINNER		
Beans & Greens Salad (Day 23 Recipe - page 129)	260	
Whole-grain bread (1 slice)	70	
Baked potato (medium)	100	
Fresh fruit in season (apple, plum, etc)	70	
Water	0	500 Cal
SNACK		
Kashi TLC Chewy Granola Bar	140	
Coffee or tea	10	150 Cal
		1490 Cal

Day 24 1500 Calorie Meal Plan

BREAKFAST	Calories	Totals
Fresh orange sliced	75	
Soft-boiled egg	80	
Whole-grain toast (2 slices)	140	
Coffee	10	305 Cal
SNACK		
Yogurt (6 oz, nonfat, any flavor)	90	
Coffee or tea	10	100 Cal
LUNCH		
Salad - 3 oz canned salmon, 1 tsp Evoo, onions & celery	200	
Lettuce & tomato wedges	20	
Rye bread (1 slice)	70	
Fresh fruit in season (apple, peach, etc)	70	
Diet soda or water	0	360 Cal
SNACK		
Popcorn Mini Bag	110	
Coffee or tea	10	120 Cal
DINNER		
Chicken breast (5 oz - broiled)	250	
Four bean salad (½ cup) (Day 24 Recipe - page 130)	135	
Large tossed salad with 1½ Tbsp low-cal dressing	70	
Water with lemon wedge	10	465 Cal
SNACK		
Graham crackers (3 squares)	90	
Skim milk (6 oz)	68	158 Cal
		1508 Cal

Day 25 1500 Calorie Meal Plan

BREAKFAST	Calories	Totals
Grapefruit (½)	75	
Cheerios (1 cup) + ½ cup skim milk + 15 raisins	190	
Coffee	10	275 Cal
SNACK		
Fresh fruit in season (peach, plum, etc)	70	
Coffee or tea	10	80 Cal
LUNCH		
Cottage cheese (1 cup low fat)	180	
Large tossed salad with 1½ Tbsp low-cal dressing	70	
Small whole-grain roll	80	
Hot or iced tea	10	340 Cal
SNACK		
Handful unsalted mixed nuts	100	
Coffee or tea	10	110 Cal
DINNER		
Hanger steak (Day 25 Recipe - page 131)	320	
Roasted potatoes (Day 25 Recipe)	120	
Cherry tomatoes (Day 25 Recipe)	20	
Steamed spinach (½ cup)	25	
Whole-grain bread (1 slice)	70	
Water	0	555 Cal
SNACK		
Kashi TLC Chewy Granola Bar	140	
Coffee or tea	10	150 Cal
		1510 Cal

Day 26 1500 Calorie Meal Plan

BREAKFAST	Calories	Totals
Cantaloupe (½ medium)	50	
Fried eggs (2 eggs)	160	
Whole-grain toast (2 slices)	140	
Coffee	10	360 Cal
SNACK		
Yogurt (6 oz, nonfat, any flavor)	90	
Coffee or tea	10	100 Cal
LUNCH		
Soup (Appendix B - page 202)	160	
Hard whole-grain roll (medium)	80	
Lettuce & tomato slices	20	
Hot or iced tea	10	270 Cal
SNACK		
Fresh fruit in season (apple, peach, etc)	70	
Coffee or tea	10	80 Cal
DINNER		
Grilled scallops (Day 26 Recipe - page 132)	210	
Grilled polenta (Day 26 Recipe)	125	
Mushroom-steamed green beans-red onion	45	
Grilled asparagus	10	
Large tossed salad with 1½ Tbsp low-cal dressing	70	
Water with lemon wedge	10	470 Cal
SNACK		
Graham crackers (4 squares)	120	
Skim milk (8 oz)	90	210 Cal
		1490 Cal

Day 27 1500 Calorie Meal Plan

BREAKFAST	Calories	Totals
Orange juice (½ cup)	50	
Oatmeal (½ cup dry) + ½ cup skim milk + 15 raisins	220	
Coffee	10	280 Cal
SNACK		
Fresh fruit in season (apple, peach, etc)	70	
Coffee or tea	10	80 Cal
LUNCH		
Two servings (1 cup) left over Day 24 bean salad	270	
Small whole-grain roll	80	
Lettuce & tomato slices	20	
Hot or iced tea	10	380 Cal
SNACK		
Yogurt (6 oz, nonfat, any flavor)	90	
Coffee or tea	10	100 Cal
DINNER		
Fettuccine (Day 27 Recipe - page 133)	290	
Large tossed salad with 1½ Tbsp low-cal dressing	70	
Italian or French bread (1 slice)	80	
Glass of red wine (4 oz)	100	
Water	0	540 Cal
SNACK		
100-Calorie Pack Cookies*	100	
Coffee or tea	10	110 Cal
* For example, Nabisco Oreo/Chips Ahoy/etc		1510 Cal

Day 28 1500 Calorie Meal Plan

BREAKFAST	Calories	Totals
Cantaloupe (½ medium)	50	
Smoothie (Day 14 Recipe - page 120)	220	
Coffee	10	280 Cal
SNACK		
Handful unsalted mixed nuts	100	
Coffee or tea	10	110 Cal
LUNCH		
Roast beef (2 oz) sandwich on whole-grain bread	295	
Lettuce	0	
Fresh fruit in season (pear, plum, etc)	70	
Hot or iced tea	10	375 Cal
SNACK		
Kashi TLC Chewy Granola Bar	140	
Coffee or tea	10	150 Cal
DINNER		
Frozen chicken dinner (Day 28 Recipe - page 134)	300	
Large tossed salad with 1½ Tbsp low-cal dressing	70	
Yogurt (6 oz, nonfat, any flavor)	90	
Water with lemon wedge	10	470 Cal
SNACK		
Popcorn Mini Bag	110	
Coffee or tea	10	120 Cal
		1505 Cal

Day 29 1500 Calorie Meal Plan

BREAKFAST	Calories	Totals
Orange juice (½ cup)	50	
Wild blueberry pancakes (Day 10 Recipe - page 116)	190	
Turkey bacon (2 slices)	70	
Light syrup (2 Tbsp)	60	
Coffee	10	380 Cal
SNACK		
Yogurt (6 oz, nonfat, any flavor)	90	
Coffee or tea	10	100 Cal
LUNCH		
Salad (3 oz canned tuna, 1 tsp Evoo, onions, celery)	175	
Lettuce & tomato wedges	20	
Rye bread (1 slice)	70	
Fresh fruit in season (apple, pear, etc)	70	
Coffee or tea	10	345 Cal
SNACK		
Handful unsalted mixed nuts	100	
Coffee or tea	10	110 Cal
DINNER		
Barbequed shrimp (Day 29 Recipe - page 135)	160	
Corn on the cob (medium)	90	
Steamed broccoli (1 cup – after cooking)	50	
Whole-grain bread (1 slice)	70	
Water	0	370 Cal
SNACK		
Graham crackers (4 squares)	120	
Skim milk (6 oz)	70	190 Cal
		1495 Cal

Day 30 1500 Calorie Meal Plan

BREAKFAST	Calories	Totals
Fresh orange sliced	75	
Kashi GoLean (1 cup) + ½ cup skim milk + ½ banana	235	
Coffee	10	320 Cal
SNACK		
Fresh fruit in season (apple, plum, etc)	70	
Coffee or tea	10	80 Cal
LUNCH		
Soup (Appendix B - page 202)	140	
Small whole-grain roll	80	
Raw zucchini slices, celery and carrot sticks	20	
Canned pineapple (½ cup, no-sugar-added)	40	
Hot or iced tea	10	290 Cal
SNACK		
Graham crackers (4 squares)	120	
Coffee or tea	10	130 Cal
DINNER		
Cheeseburger (Day 30 Recipe - page 136)	370	
Lettuce and sliced tomato	20	
Whole-grain hard roll	140	
Steamed green beans	25	
Pickle spear	0	
Water with lemon wedge	10	565 Cal
SNACK		
Popcorn Mini Bag	110	
Coffee or tea	10	120 Cal
		1505 Cal

Day 31 1500 Calorie Meal Plan

BREAKFAST	Calories	Totals
Grapefruit (½)	75	
Scrambled egg	80	
Turkey bacon (1 slice)	35	
Whole-grain toast (1 slice)	70	
Coffee	10	270 Cal
SNACK		
Yogurt (6 oz, nonfat, any flavor)	90	
Coffee or tea	10	100 Cal
LUNCH		
Ham (2 oz) with mustard on 2 slices rye bread	300	
Pickle spear	0	
Small bunch of grapes	65	
Gelatin dessert (unsweetened)	10	
Hot or iced tea	10	385 Cal
SNACK		
Fresh fruit in season (apple, plum, etc)	70	
Coffee or tea	10	80 Cal
DINNER		
Baked Sea Bass (Day 31 Recipe - page 137)	395	
Large tossed salad with 1½ Tbsp low-cal dressing	70	
Water with lemon wedge	10	475 Cal
SNACK		
100-Calorie Pack Cookies	100	
Skim milk (8 oz)	90	190 Cal
		1500 Cal

46

Day 32 1500 Calorie Meal Plan

BREAKFAST	Calories	Totals
Grapefruit (½)	75	
Cheerios (1 cup) + ½ cup skim milk + about 15 raisins	190	
Coffee	10	275 Cal
SNACK		
Fresh fruit in season (pear, plum, etc)	70	
Coffee or tea	10	80 Cal
LUNCH		
Subway 6" (Turkey Breast, Cheese + veggies)*	230	
Tossed salad with 1½ Tbsp low-cal dressing	70	
Hot or iced tea	10	310 Cal
SNACK		
Handful unsalted mixed nuts	100	
Coffee or tea	10	110 Cal
DINNER		
Turkey & veggies (Day 32 Recipe - page 138)	350	
Spinach (½ cup steamed & drizzled with 1 tsp	70	
Romaine lettuce, tomato slices & 1 Tbsp low-cal dressing	45	
Whole-grain bread (1 slice)	70	
Water	0	535 Cal
SNACK		
Two small cookies	160	
Coffee or tea	10	170 Cal
* On 6" half wheat roll.		1480 Cal

Day 33 1500 Calorie Meal Plan

BREAKFAST	Calories	Totals
Cantaloupe (½ medium)	50	
Fried egg	80	
Turkey bacon (1 slice)	35	
Toasted raisin bread (1 slice)	75	
Coffee	10	250 Cal
SNACK		
Yogurt (6 oz, nonfat, any flavor)	90	
Coffee or tea	10	100 Cal
LUNCH		
Steak, Egg & Cheese*	280	
Canned pineapple (½ cup, no sugar added)	40	
Diet soda or water	0	320 Cal
* Hot Pockets (wrap)		
SNACK		
Dark chocolate (1 oz)	150	150 Cal
DINNER		
Frozen fish dinner (Day 33 Recipe - page 139)	340	
Large tossed salad with 1½ Tbsp low-cal dressing	70	
Whole-grain bread (1 slice)	70	
Fresh fruit in season (peach, plum, etc)	70	
Water with lemon wedge	10	560 Cal
SNACK		
Popcorn Mini Bag	110	
Coffee or tea	10	120 Cal
		1495 Cal

Day 34 1500 Calorie Meal Plan

BREAKFAST	Calories	Totals
Tomato juice (½ cup)	20	
Shredded Wheat (1 cup) + ½ cup skim milk + ½ banana	265	
Coffee	10	295 Cal
SNACK		
Handful unsalted mixed nuts	100	
Coffee or tea	10	110 Cal
LUNCH		
Roast beef (2 oz) with lettuce sandwich	300	
Hot or iced tea	10	310 Cal
SNACK		
Carrot sticks + ¼ cup low-fat cottage cheese & chives	60	
Coffee or tea	10	70 Cal
DINNER		
Pasta Rapini (Day 34 Recipe - page 140)	290	
Large tossed green salad with 1½ Tbsp low-cal	70	
Fresh fruit in season (apple, peach, etc)	70	
Italian or French bread (1 slice)	80	
Glass of red wine (4 oz)	100	
Water	0	610 Cal
SNACK		
Graham Crackers (3 squares)	90	
Coffee or tea	10	100 Cal
		1495 Cal

Day 35 1500 Calorie Meal Plan

BREAKFAST	Calories	Totals
Cantaloupe (½ medium)	50	
Oatmeal (½ cup dry) + ½ cup skim milk + about 15 raisins	220	
Coffee	10	280 Cal
SNACK		
Fresh fruit in season (apple, peach, etc)	70	
Coffee or tea	10	80 Cal
LUNCH		
Soup (**Appendix B** - page 202)	90	
Grilled cheese sandwich (2 slices 2% American	240	
Lettuce and sliced tomato	20	
Pickle spear	0	
Water	0	350 Cal
SNACK		
Carrot sticks + ¼ cup low-fat cottage cheese & chives	60	60 Cal
DINNER		
Eat Out – Chicken dinner (**Day 35 Recipe** - page 141)		
Max allowable calories	630	630 Cal
SNACK		
100-Calorie Pack Cookies	100	
Coffee or tea	10	110 Cal
		1510 Cal

Day 36 1500 Calorie Meal Plan

BREAKFAST	Calories	Totals
Cantaloupe (½ medium)	50	
Wheaties (¾ cup) + ½ cup skim milk + ½ banana	190	
Whole-grain toast (1 slice)	70	
Coffee	10	320 Cal
SNACK		
Fresh fruit in season (apple, pear, etc)	70	
Coffee or tea	10	80 Cal
LUNCH		
Chicken, Broccoli & Cheese*	270	
Diet soda or water	0	270 Cal
* Hot Pockets (wrap)		
SNACK		
Kashi TLC Chewy Granola Bar	140	
Coffee or tea	10	150 Cal
DINNER		
Grilled Tilapia (Day 36 Recipe - page 142)	300	
Asparagus spear (6)	25	
Wild rice (½ cup – after cooking)	100	
Large tossed salad with 1½ Tbsp low-cal dressing	70	
Water with lemon wedge	10	505 Cal
SNACK		
100-Calorie Pack Cookies	100	
Skim milk (6 oz)	70	170 Cal
		1495 Cal

Day 37 1500 Calorie Meal Plan

BREAKFAST	Calories	Totals
Orange juice (½ cup)	50	
Soft-boiled egg	80	
Whole-grain toast (2 slices)	140	
Coffee	10	280 Cal
SNACK		
Yogurt (6 oz, nonfat, any flavor)	90	
Coffee or tea	10	100 Cal
LUNCH		
Salad (3 oz canned tuna, 1 tsp Evoo, onions, celery)	175	
Lettuce & tomato wedges + rye bread (1 slice)	90	
Fresh fruit in season – (apple, pear, etc)	70	
Gelatin dessert (unsweetened)	10	
Hot or iced tea	10	355 Cal
SNACK		
Handful unsalted mixed nuts	100	
Coffee or tea	10	110 Cal
DINNER		
Low-Cal Beef Stew (Day 37 Recipe - page 143)	365	
Large tossed salad with 1½ Tbsp low-cal dressing	70	
Small whole-grain roll	80	
Water with lemon wedge	10	525 Cal
SNACK		
Graham crackers (4 squares)	120	
Coffee or tea	10	130 Cal
		1500 Cal

Day 38 1500 Calorie Meal Plan

BREAKFAST	Calories	Totals
Cantaloupe (½ medium)	50	
Smoothie (Day 14 Recipe - page 120)	220	
Coffee	10	280 Cal
SNACK		
Popcorn Mini Bag	110	
Coffee or tea	10	120 Cal
LUNCH		
Peanut butter (2 Tbsp) on 2 slices whole-grain bread	340	
Skim milk (6 oz)	70	
Fresh fruit in season (apple, plum, etc)	70	480 Cal
SNACK		
Coffee or tea	10	10 Cal
DINNER		
Pan-broiled lamb chop (Day 38 Recipe - page 144)	320	
Large tossed salad with 1½ Tbsp low-cal dressing	70	
Small whole-grain roll	80	
Water with lemon wedge	10	480 Cal
SNACK		
100-Calorie Pack Cookies	100	
Coffee or tea	10	110 Cal
		1490 Cal

Day 39 1500 Calorie Meal Plan

BREAKFAST	Calories	Totals
Fresh sliced orange	75	
Cheerios (1 cup) + ½ cup skim milk + about 15 raisins	190	
Whole grain toast (1 slice)	70	
Coffee	10	345 Cal
SNACK		
Fresh fruit in season (peach, plum, etc)	70	
Coffee or tea	10	80 Cal
LUNCH		
Cottage cheese (1 cup low fat)	180	
Large tossed salad with 1½ Tbsp low-cal dressing	70	
Small whole-grain roll	80	
Hot or iced tea	10	340 Cal
SNACK		
Handful unsalted mixed nuts	100	
Coffee or tea	10	110 Cal
DINNER		
Chicken with veggies (Day 39 Recipe - page 145)	365	
Yogurt (6 oz nonfat, any flavor)	90	
Water with lemon wedge	10	465 Cal
SNACK		
Dark chocolate (1 oz)	150	
Coffee or tea	10	160 Cal
		1500 Cal

54

Day 40 1500 Calorie Meal Plan

BREAKFAST	Calories	Totals
Grapefruit (½)	75	
Scrambled egg	80	
Turkey bacon (2 slices)	70	
Toasted raisin bread (1 slice)	75	
Coffee	10	310 Cal
SNACK		
Yogurt (6 oz, nonfat, any flavor)	90	
Coffee or tea	10	100 Cal
LUNCH		
Soup (Appendix B - page 202)	150	
Large tossed salad with 1½ Tbsp low-cal dressing	70	
Whole-grain bread (1 slice)	70	
Hot or iced tea	10	300 Cal
SNACK		
Fresh fruit in season (apple, plum, etc)	70	
Coffee or tea	10	80 Cal
DINNER		
Eat Out – Fish dinner (Day 40 Recipe - page 146)		
Max allowable calories	595	595 Cal
SNACK		
Skinny Cow Low-Fat Fudge Bar	100	
Coffee or tea	10	110 Cal
		1495 Cal

Day 41 1500 Calorie Meal Plan

BREAKFAST	Calories	Totals
Orange juice (½ cup)	50	
Shredded Wheat (1 cup) + ½ cup skim milk + ½ banana	260	
Coffee	10	320 Cal
SNACK		
Handful unsalted mixed nuts	100	
Coffee or tea	10	110 Cal
LUNCH		
Turkey frank (2 oz) with mustard & relish	150	
Hot dog bun	130	
Diet soda	0	280 Cal
SNACK		
Yogurt (6 oz, nonfat, any flavor)	90	
Coffee or tea	10	100 Cal
DINNER		
Pasta e Fagioli (Day 41 Recipe - page 147)	300	
Large tossed salad with 1½ Tbsp low-cal dressing	70	
Italian or French bread (1 slice)	80	
Glass of red wine (4 oz)	100	
Water with lemon wedge	10	560 Cal
SNACK		
Graham crackers (4 squares)	120	
Coffee or tea	10	130 Cal
		1500 Cal

Day 42 1500 Calorie Meal Plan

BREAKFAST	Calories	Totals
Cantaloupe (½ medium)	50	
Wheaties (¾ cup) + ½ cup skim milk + ½ banana	190	
Coffee	10	250 Cal
SNACK		
Handful unsalted mixed nuts	100	
Coffee or tea	10	110 Cal
LUNCH		
Grilled Swiss cheese sandwich (2 oz low-fat cheese)	310	
Pickle spear	0	
Hot or iced tea	10	320 Cal
SNACK		
Dark chocolate (1 oz)	150	
Coffee or tea	10	160 Cal
DINNER		
Frozen chicken dinner (Day 28 Recipe - page 134)	300	
Large tossed salad with 1½ Tbsp low-cal dressing	70	
Fresh fruit in season (peach, plum, etc)	70	
Water	0	450 Cal
SNACK		
Blueberry Muffin (Day 42 Recipe - page 148)	145	
Skim milk (6 oz)	65	210 Cal
		1500 Cal

Day 43 1500 Calorie Meal Plan

BREAKFAST	Calories	Totals
Fresh or frozen strawberries (½ cup)	25	
French toasted English Muffin (Day 3 Recipe - page 148)	270	
Light syrup (1 Tbsp)	30	
Coffee	10	335 Cal
SNACK		
Yogurt (6 oz, nonfat, any flavor)	90	
Coffee or tea	10	100 Cal
LUNCH		
Salad (3 oz canned tuna, 1 tsp Evoo, onions, celery)	175	
Lettuce & tomato wedges	20	
Rye bread (1 slice)	70	
Coffee or tea	10	275 Cal
SNACK		
Handful unsalted mixed nuts	100	
Coffee or tea	10	110 Cal
DINNER		
Beef Kebob with veggies (Day 43 Recipe - page 149)	390	
Baked potato (medium)	100	
Fresh fruit in season (apple, pear, etc)	70	
Water	0	560 Cal
SNACK		
Graham crackers (4 squares)	120	
Coffee or tea	10	130 Cal
		1510 Cal

Day 44 1500 Calorie Meal Plan

BREAKFAST	Calories	Totals
Orange juice (½ cup)	50	
Kashi GoLean (1 cup) + ½ cup skim milk + ½ banana	235	
Coffee	10	295 Cal
SNACK		
Fresh fruit in season (pear, peach, etc)	70	
Coffee or tea	10	80 Cal
LUNCH		
Soup (Appendix B - page 202)	100	
Small whole-grain roll	80	
Lettuce and sliced tomato with 1 Tbsp low-cal	45	
Unsweetened apple sauce (½ cup)	45	
Hot or iced tea	10	280 Cal
SNACK		
Popcorn Mini Bag	110	
Coffee or tea	10	120 Cal
DINNER		
Baked Haddock (Day 44 Recipe - page 150)	420	
Large tossed salad with 1½ Tbsp low-cal dressing	70	
Yogurt (6 oz, nonfat, any flavor)	90	
Water	0	580 Cal
SNACK		
Skinny Cow Ice Cream Sandwich	140	
Coffee or tea	10	150 Cal
		1505 Cal

Day 45 1500 Calorie Meal Plan

BREAKFAST	Calories	Totals
Orange juice (½ cup)	50	
Fried egg	80	
Toasted raisin bread (1 slice)	75	
Coffee	10	215 Cal
SNACK		
Yogurt (6 oz, nonfat, any flavor)	90	
Coffee or tea	10	100 Cal
LUNCH		
Chicken, Bacon Ranch*	270	
Small bunch of grapes	50	
Diet soda or water	0	320 Cal
* Hot Pockets (wrap)		
SNACK		
Handful unsalted mixed nuts	100	
Coffee or tea	10	110 Cal
DINNER		
Chicken Cacciatore (Day 45 Recipe - page 151)	310	
Italian or French bread (1 slice)	80	
Glass of red wine (4 oz)	100	
Fresh fruit in season (apple, peach, etc)	70	
Water	0	560 Cal
SNACK		
Blueberry muffin	145	
Coffee or tea	10	155 Cal
		1490 Cal

<u>Day 46</u> 1500 Calorie Meal Plan

BREAKFAST	Calories	Totals
Grapefruit (½)	75	
Cheerios (1 cup) + ½ cup skim milk + about 15 raisins	190	
Coffee	10	275 Cal
SNACK		
Fresh fruit in season (apple, peach, etc)	70	
Coffee or tea	10	80 Cal
LUNCH		
Subway 6" (Ham, Cheese + veggies)*	260	
Large tossed salad with 1½ Tbsp low-cal dressing	70	
Hot or iced tea	10	340 Cal
SNACK		
Handful unsalted mixed nuts	100	
Coffee or tea	10	110 Cal
DINNER		
Poached Cod (Day 46 Recipe - page 152)	275	
Grilled potatoes	100	
Grilled cherry tomatoes	45	
Spinach (½ cup) steamed with garlic & drizzled	50	
Whole-grain bread (1 slice)	70	
Water with lemon wedge	10	550 Cal
SNACK		
Blueberry muffin	145	
Coffee or tea	10	155 Cal
* On 6" half wheat roll.		1510 Cal

Day 47 1500 Calorie Meal Plan

BREAKFAST	Calories	Totals
Grapefruit (½)	75	
Scrambled egg	80	
Whole grain toast (1 slice)	70	
Coffee	10	235 Cal
SNACK		
Handful unsalted mixed nuts	100	
Coffee or tea	10	110 Cal
LUNCH		
Soup (Appendix B - page 202)	110	
Turkey (1 oz) on 1 slice of rye bread (½ sandwich)	115	
Lettuce & tomato slices	20	
Hot or iced tea	10	235 Cal
SNACK		
Fresh fruit in season (peach, plum, etc)	70	
Coffee or tea	10	80 Cal
DINNER		
Eat Out – Chinese food (Day 19 Recipe - page 125)		
Max allowable calories	640	640 Cal
SNACK		
Graham crackers (4 squares)	120	
Skim milk (6 oz)	70	190 Cal
		1490 Cal

Day 48 1500 Calorie Meal Plan

BREAKFAST	Calories	Totals
Cantaloupe (½ medium)	50	
Smoothie (Day 14 Recipe - page 120)	220	
Coffee	10	280 Cal
SNACK		
Handful unsalted mixed nuts	100	
Coffee or tea	10	110 Cal
LUNCH		
Left over Chinese food from Day 47	260	
Gelatin dessert (unsweetened)	10	
Hot or iced tea	10	280 Cal
SNACK		
Yogurt (6 oz, nonfat, any flavor)	90	
Coffee or tea	10	100 Cal
DINNER		
Pasta Salad (Day 48 Recipe - page 154)	370	
Italian or French bread (1 slice)	80	
Glass of red wine (4 oz)	100	
Water with lemon wedge	10	560 Cal
SNACK		
Blueberry muffin	145	
Coffee or tea	10	155 Cal
		1485 Cal

63

Day 49 1500 Calorie Meal Plan

BREAKFAST	Calories	Totals
Cantaloupe (½ medium)	50	
Oatmeal (½ cup dry) + ½ cup skim milk + about 15 raisins	220	
Coffee	10	280 Cal
SNACK		
Handful unsalted mixed nuts	100	
Coffee or tea	10	110 Cal
LUNCH		
Turkey breast (2 oz) on 2 slices whole-grain bread	245	
Lettuce, tomato and 1 Tbsp light mayo	35	
Pickle spear	0	
Fresh fruit in season (apple, plum, etc)	70	
Hot or iced tea	10	360 Cal
SNACK		
Graham crackers (3 squares)	90	
Skim milk (6 oz)	65	155 Cal
DINNER		
Frozen meat dinner (Day 21 Recipe - page 127)	300	
Large tossed salad with 1½ Tbsp low-cal dressing	70	
Whole-grain bread (1 slice)	70	
Water with lemon wedge	10	450 Cal
SNACK		
Blueberry muffin	145	
Coffee or tea	10	155 Cal
		1510 Cal

Day 50 1500 Calorie Meal Plan

BREAKFAST	Calories	Totals
Fresh or frozen strawberries (1 cup)	25	
French toasted English Muffin (Day 3 Recipe page 109)	270	
Light syrup (1 Tbsp)	30	
Coffee	10	335 Cal
SNACK		
Fresh fruit in season (pear, plum, etc)	70	
Coffee or tea	10	80 Cal
LUNCH		
Soup (Appendix B - page 202)	120	
BLT sandwich (2 slices turkey bacon, 1 Tbsp light	245	
Pickle spear	0	
Diet soda or water	0	365 Cal
SNACK		
Popcorn Mini Bag	110	
Coffee or tea	10	120 Cal
DINNER		
Pan-fried Sole (Day 50 Recipe - page 156)	325	
Large tossed salad with 1½ Tbsp low-cal dressing	70	
Whole-grain bread (1 slice)	70	
Water	0	465 Cal
SNACK		
Skinny Cow Ice Cream Sandwich	140	140 Cal
		1505 Cal

Day 51 1500 Calorie Meal Plan

BREAKFAST	Calories	Totals
Orange juice (½ cup)	50	
Wheaties (¾ cup) + ½ cup skim milk + ½ banana	190	
Whole-grain toast (1 slice)	70	
Coffee	10	320 Cal
SNACK		
Handful unsalted mixed nuts	100	
Coffee or tea	10	110 Cal
LUNCH		
Ham (2 oz) with mustard on 2 slices rye bread	290	
Pickle spear	0	
Small bunch of grapes	65	
Hot or iced tea	10	365 Cal
SNACK		
Yogurt (6 oz, nonfat, any flavor)	90	
Coffee or tea	10	100 Cal
DINNER		
Beans and Greens Salad (Day 51 Recipe - page 157)	260	
Whole-grain bread (1 slice)	70	
Baked potato (medium)	100	
Fresh fruit in season (apple, peach, etc)	70	
Water	0	500 Cal
SNACK		
100-Calorie Pack Cookies	100	
Coffee or tea	10	110 Cal
		1505 Cal

Day 52 1500 Calorie Meal Plan

BREAKFAST	Calories	Totals
Fresh orange sliced	75	
Soft-boiled egg	80	
Whole grain toast (2 slices)	140	
Coffee	10	305 Cal
SNACK		
Yogurt (6 oz, nonfat, any flavor)	90	
Coffee or tea	10	100 Cal
LUNCH		
Salad – 3 oz canned salmon, 1 tsp Evoo, onions & celery	200	
Lettuce & tomato wedges	20	
Rye bread (1 slice)	70	
Fresh fruit in season (apple, peach, etc)	70	
Coffee or tea	10	370 Cal
AFTERNOON SNACK		
Handful unsalted mixed nuts	100	
Coffee or tea	10	110 Cal
DINNER		
Chicken Piccata (Day 52 Recipe - page 158)	270	
Brown rice (½ cup – after cooking)	100	
Large tossed salad with 1½ Tbsp low-cal dressing	70	
Water with lemon wedge	10	450 Cal
SNACK		
Graham crackers (4 squares)	120	
Skim milk (4 oz)	45	165 Cal
		1500 Cal

Day 53 1500 Calorie Meal Plan

BREAKFAST	Calories	Totals
Grapefruit (½)	75	
Cheerios (1 cup) + ½ cup skim milk + about 15 raisins	190	
Coffee	10	275 Cal
SNACK		
Fresh fruit in season (peach, plum, etc)	70	
Coffee or tea	10	80 Cal
LUNCH		
Cottage cheese (1 cup low fat)	180	
Large tossed salad with 1½ Tbsp low-cal dressing	70	
Small whole-grain roll	80	
Hot or iced tea	10	340 Cal
SNACK		
Handful unsalted mixed nuts	100	
Coffee or tea	10	110 Cal
DINNER		
Beef steak strips (Day 53 Recipe - page 159)	330	
Steamed spinach (½ cup)	25	
Baked potato (medium)	100	
Whole-grain bread (1 slice)	70	
Water with lemon wedge	10	535 Cal
SNACK		
Blueberry muffin	145	
Coffee or tea	10	155 Cal
		1495 Cal

Day 54 1500 Calorie Meal Plan

BREAKFAST	Calories	Totals
Orange juice (½ cup)	50	
Fried eggs (2 eggs)	160	
Toasted whole-grain bread (2 slices)	140	
Coffee	10	360 Cal
SNACK		
Yogurt (6 oz, nonfat, any flavor)	90	
Coffee or tea	10	100 Cal
LUNCH		
Soup (Appendix B - page 202)	200	
Small whole-grain roll	80	
Lettuce & tomato slices	20	
Hot or iced tea	10	310 Cal
SNACK		
Fresh fruit in season (pear, plum, etc)	70	
Coffee or tea	10	80 Cal
DINNER		
Grilled scallops (Day 54 Recipe - page 160)	210	
Grilled polenta (Day 54 Recipe)	125	
Mushroom-steamed green beans-red onion (Day 54)	45	
Grilled asparagus (Day 54)	10	
Large tossed salad with 1½ Tbsp low-cal dressing	70	
Water with lemon wedge	10	470 Cal
SNACK		
Graham crackers (4 squares)	120	
Skim milk (6 oz)	65	185 Cal
		1505 Cal

Day 55 1500 Calorie Meal Plan

BREAKFAST	Calories	Totals
Cantaloupe (½ medium)	50	
Oatmeal (½ cup dry) + ½ cup skim milk + about 15 raisins	220	
Coffee	10	280 Cal
SNACK		
Fresh fruit in season (apple, plum, etc)	70	
Coffee or tea	10	80 Cal
LUNCH		
Two servings (1 cup) left over Day 51 bean salad	270	
Small whole-grain roll	80	
Lettuce & tomato slices	20	
Hot or iced tea	10	380 Cal
SNACK		
Celery sticks + ¼ cup low-fat cottage cheese & chives	60	
Coffee or tea	10	70 Cal
DINNER		
Hearty Vegetable Soup (Day 55 Recipe - page 161)	360	
Large tossed salad with 1½ Tbsp low-cal dressing	70	
Italian or French bread (1 slice)	80	
Water with lemon wedge	10	520 Cal
SNACK		
Blueberry muffin	145	
Coffee or tea	10	155 Cal
		1485 Cal

Day 56 1500 Calorie Meal Plan

BREAKFAST	Calories	Totals
Tomato juice (½ cup)	20	
Shredded Wheat (1 cup) + ½ cup skim milk + ½ banana	260	
Coffee	10	290 Cal
SNACK		
Handful unsalted mixed nuts	100	
Coffee or tea	10	110 Cal
LUNCH		
Roast beef (2 oz) sandwich on whole-grain bread	305	
Lettuce	0	
Fresh fruit in season (peach, plum, etc)	70	
Hot or iced tea	10	385 Cal
SNACK		
Yogurt (6 oz, nonfat, any flavor)	90	
Coffee or tea	10	100 Cal
DINNER		
Frozen chicken dinner (Day 28 Recipe - page 134)	300	
Large tossed salad with 1½ Tbsp low-cal dressing	70	
Whole-grain bread (1 slice)	70	
Water with lemon wedge	10	450 Cal
SNACK		
Graham crackers (4 squares)	120	
Skim milk (4 oz)	45	165 Cal
		1500 Cal

Day 57 1500 Calorie Meal Plan

BREAKFAST	Calories	Totals
Cantaloupe (½ medium)	50	
Smoothie (Day 14 Recipe - page 120)	220	
Coffee	10	280 Cal
SNACK		
Handful unsalted mixed nuts	100	
Coffee or tea	10	110 Cal
LUNCH		
Salad (3 oz canned tuna, 1 tsp Evoo, onions, celery)	175	
Lettuce & tomato wedges	20	
Rye bread (1 slice)	70	
Fresh fruit in season (apple, pear, etc)	70	
Coffee or tea	10	345 Cal
SNACK		
Graham crackers (3 squares)	90	
Coffee or tea	10	100 Cal
DINNER		
Salmon - Mango Salsa (Day 57 Recipe - page 163)	460	
Large tossed salad with 1½ Tbsp low-cal dressing	70	
Water	10	540 Cal
SNACK		
Skinny Cow Ice Cream Sandwich	140	140 Cal
		1505 Cal

Day 58 1500 Calorie Meal Plan

BREAKFAST	Calories	Totals
Tomato juice (½ cup)	20	
Kashi GoLean (1 cup) + ½ cup skim milk	185	
Coffee	10	265 Cal
SNACK		
Fresh fruit in season (apple, plum, etc)	70	
Coffee or tea	10	80 Cal
LUNCH		
Soup (Appendix B - page 202)	150	
Small whole-grain roll	80	
Lettuce and sliced tomato with 1 Tbsp low-cal	45	
Unsweetened apple sauce (½ cup)	45	
Hot or iced tea	10	330 Cal
SNACK		
Popcorn Mini Bag	110	
Coffee or tea	10	120 Cal
DINNER		
Grilled pork chop - orange (Day 57 Recipe - page 164)	470	
Wild rice (¼ cup – after cooking	50	
Asparagus (7 spear cooked & drained)	20	
Large tossed salad with 1½ Tbsp low-cal dressing	70	
Water	0	610 Cal
SNACK		
Blueberry muffin	145	
Coffee or tea	10	155 Cal
		1510 Cal

Day 59 1500 Calorie Meal Plan

BREAKFAST	Calories	Totals
Grapefruit (½)	75	
Scrambled egg	80	
Turkey bacon (2 slices)	70	
Whole-grain toast (1 slice)	70	
Coffee	10	305 Cal
SNACK		
Yogurt (6 oz, nonfat, any flavor)	90	
Coffee or tea	10	100 Cal
LUNCH		
Soup (Appendix B - page 202)	130	
Tomato slices ¼ cup chopped fresh basil + 1 tsp Evoo	60	
Whole-grain bread (1 slice)	70	
Gelatin dessert (unsweetened)	10	
Hot or iced tea	10	280 Cal
SNACK		
Fresh fruit in season (peach, plum, etc)	70	
Coffee or tea	10	80 Cal
DINNER		
Eat Out – Fish dinner (Day 5 Recipe - page 111)		
Max allowable calories	595	595 Cal
SNACK		
Skinny Cow Ice Cream Sandwich	140	
Coffee or tea	10	150 Cal
		1510 Cal

Day 60 1500 Calorie Meal Plan

BREAKFAST	Calories	Totals
Grapefruit (½)	75	
Cheerios (1 cup) + ½ cup skim milk + about 15 raisins	190	
Coffee	10	275 Cal
SNACK		
Fresh fruit in season (peach, plum, etc)	70	
Coffee or tea	10	80 Cal
LUNCH		
Subway 6" (Ham, Cheese + veggies)*	260	
Large tossed salad with 1½ Tbsp low-cal dressing	70	
Hot or iced tea	10	340 Cal
SNACK		
Handful unsalted mixed nuts	100	
Coffee or tea	10	110 Cal
DINNER		
Chicken Stew (Day 60 Recipe - page 166)	360	
Brown rice (½ cup – after cooking)	100	
Small whole-grain roll	80	
Water	0	540 Cal
SNACK		
Kashi TLC Chewy Granola Bar	140	
Coffee or tea	10	150 Cal
		1495 Cal

Day 61 1500 Calorie Meal Plan

BREAKFAST	Calories	Totals
Orange juice (½ cup)	50	
Wheaties (¾ cup) + ½ cup skim milk + ½ banana	190	
Whole-grain toast (1 slice)	70	
Coffee	10	320 Cal
SNACK		
Fresh fruit in season (pear, peach, etc)	70	
Coffee or tea	10	80 Cal
LUNCH		
Soup (Appendix B - page 202)	160	
Turkey breast (1 oz) on 1 slice rye bread	105	
Pickle spear	0	
Hot or iced tea	10	275 Cal
SNACK		
Popcorn Mini Bag	110	
Coffee or tea	10	120 Cal
DINNER		
Shrimp over Spaghetti (Day 61 Recipe - page 167)	450	
Large tossed salad with 1½ Tbsp low-cal dressing	70	
Water with lemon wedge	10	530 Cal
SNACK		
Graham crackers (4 squares)	120	
Skim milk (6 oz)	70	190 Cal
		1515 Cal

Day 62 1500 Calorie Meal Plan

BREAKFAST	Calories	Totals
Fresh or frozen strawberries (½ cup)	25	
French toasted English Muffin (Day 3 Recipe - page 109)	270	
Light syrup (1 Tbsp)	30	
Coffee	10	335 Cal
SNACK		
Yogurt (6 oz, nonfat, any flavor)	90	
Coffee or tea	10	100 Cal
LUNCH		
Salad (3 oz canned tuna, 1 tsp Evoo, onions, celery)	175	
Lettuce & tomato wedges	20	
Rye bread (1 slice)	70	
Fresh fruit in season (apple, pear, etc)	70	
Coffee or tea	10	345 Cal
SNACK		
Handful unsalted mixed nuts	100	
Coffee or tea	10	110 Cal
DINNER		
Beef Burgundy (Day 62 Recipe - page 168)	350	
Large tossed salad with 1½ Tbsp low-cal dressing	70	
Whole-grain bread (1 slice)	70	
Water	0	490 Cal
SNACK		
Popcorn Mini Bag	110	
Coffee or tea	10	120 Cal
		1500 Cal

Day 63 1500 Calorie Meal Plan

BREAKFAST	Calories	Totals
Grapefruit (½)	75	
Scrambled egg	80	
Turkey bacon (1 slice)	35	
Whole grain toast (1 slice)	70	
Coffee	10	270 Cal
SNACK		
Yogurt (6 oz nonfat, any flavor)	90	
Coffee or tea	10	100 Cal
LUNCH		
Ham (2 oz) with mustard on 2 slices rye bread	290	
Pickle spear	0	
Gelatin dessert (unsweetened)	10	
Hot or iced tea	10	310 Cal
SNACK		
Fresh fruit in season (peach, plum, etc)	70	
Coffee or tea	10	80 Cal
DINNER		
Chicken cutlet (Day 63 Recipe - page 169)	450	
Two small baked potatoes	100	
Large tossed salad with 1½ Tbsp low-cal dressing*	70	
Water with lemon wedge	10	630 Cal
* Day 63 recipe shows much of salad on plate with cutlet.		
SNACK		
Skinny Cow Low Fat Fudge Bar	100	
Coffee or tea	10	110 Cal
		1500 Cal

Day 64 1500 Calorie Meal Plan

BREAKFAST	Calories	Totals
Grapefruit (½)	75	
Cheerios (1 cup) + ½ cup skim milk + about 15 raisins	190	
Coffee	10	275 Cal
SNACK		
Fresh fruit in season (apple, plum, etc)	70	
Coffee or tea	10	80 Cal
LUNCH		
Cottage cheese (1 cup low fat)	180	
Tossed salad with 1½ Tbsp low-cal dressing	70	
Small whole-grain roll	80	
Hot or iced tea	10	340 Cal
SNACK		
Handful unsalted mixed nuts	100	
Coffee or tea	10	110 Cal
DINNER		
Personal-Size Meat Loaf (Day 64 Recipe - page 170)	410	
Brown rice (½ cup – after cooking)	100	
Green beans - steamed	30	
Water	0	540 Cal
SNACK		
Blueberry muffin	145	
Coffee or tea	10	155 Cal
		1500 Cal

Day 65 1500 Calorie Meal Plan

BREAKFAST	Calories	Totals
Cantaloupe (½ medium)	50	
Smoothie (Day 14 Recipe - page 120)	220	
Coffee	10	280 Cal
SNACK		
Popcorn Mini Bag	110	
Coffee or tea	10	120 Cal
LUNCH		
Soup (Appendix B - page 202)	130	
Small whole-grain roll	80	
Lettuce and sliced tomato with 1 Tbsp low-cal	45	
Canned pineapple (½ cup, no-sugar-added juice)	40	
Hot or iced tea	10	305 Cal
SNACK		
Yogurt (6 oz, nonfat, any flavor)	90	
Coffee or tea	10	100 Cal
DINNER		
Frozen fish dinner (Day 5 Recipe - page 111)	340	
Large tossed salad with 1½ Tbsp low-cal dressing	70	
Whole-grain bread (1 slice)	70	
Fresh fruit in season (apple, pear, etc)	70	
Water with lemon wedge	10	560 Cal
SNACK		
Kashi TLC Chewy Granola Bar	140	140 Cal
		1495 Cal

Day 66 1500 Calorie Meal Plan

BREAKFAST	Calories	Totals
Tomato juice (½ cup)	20	
Shredded Wheat (1 cup) + ½ cup skim milk + ½ banana	265	
Coffee	10	295 Cal
SNACK		
Handful unsalted mixed nuts	100	
Coffee or tea	10	110 Cal
LUNCH		
Left over meat loaf (½ of Day 64 serving)	205	
Small whole-grain roll	80	
Lettuce	0	
Hot or iced tea	10	295 Cal
SNACK		
Yogurt (6 oz, nonfat, any flavor)	90	
Coffee or tea	10	100 Cal
DINNER		
Pita Pizza (Day 66 Recipe - page 172)	430	
Large tossed salad with 1½ Tbsp low-cal dressing	70	
Glass red wine (4 oz)	100	
Water	0	600 Cal
SNACK		
100-Calorie Pack Cookies	100	
Coffee or tea	10	110 Cal
		1510 Cal

Day 67 1500 Calorie Meal Plan

BREAKFAST	Calories	Totals
Cantaloupe (½ medium)	50	
Oatmeal (½ cup dry) + ½ cup skim milk + about 15 raisins	220	
Coffee	10	280 Cal
SNACK		
Fresh fruit in season (apple, plum, etc)	70	
Coffee or tea	10	80 Cal
LUNCH		
Subway 6" (Ham, Cheese + veggies)*	260	
Large tossed salad with 1½ Tbsp low-cal dressing	70	
Hot or iced tea	10	340 Cal
SNACK		
Carrot sticks + ¼ cup low-fat cottage cheese & chives	60	
Coffee or tea	10	70 Cal
DINNER		
Eat Out – Chicken (Day 7 Recipe - page 113)		
Max allowable calories	630	630 Cal
SNACK		
Skinny Cow Low Fat Fudge Bar	100	
Coffee or tea	10	110 Cal
		1510 Cal

Day 68 1500 Calorie Meal Plan

BREAKFAST	Calories	Totals
Cantaloupe (½ medium)	50	
Wheaties (¾ cup) + ½ cup skim milk + ½ banana	190	
Whole grain toast (1 slice)	70	
Coffee	10	320 Cal
SNACK		
Fresh fruit in season (peach, plum, etc)	70	
Coffee or tea	10	80 Cal
LUNCH		
Turkey (2 oz) on 2 slices rye bread	240	
Lettuce & tomato	10	
Diet soda or water	0	250 Cal
SNACK		
Kashi TLC Chewy Granola Bar	140	
Coffee or tea	10	150 Cal
DINNER		
Pork Medallions lime sauce (Day 68 Recipe - page 174	450	
Green beans - steamed	25	
Large tossed salad with 1½ Tbsp low-cal dressing	70	
Water	0	545 Cal
SNACK		
Graham crackers (4 squares)	120	
Skim milk (4 oz)	45	165 Cal
		1505 Cal

Day 69 1500 Calorie Meal Plan

BREAKFAST	Calories	Totals
Orange juice (½ cup)	50	
Soft-boiled egg	80	
Whole grain toast (2 slices)	140	
Coffee	10	280 Cal
SNACK		
Yogurt (6 oz, nonfat, any flavor)	90	
Coffee or tea	10	100 Cal
LUNCH		
Salad (3 oz canned tuna, 1 tsp Evoo, onions, celery)	175	
Lettuce & tomato wedges + rye bread (1 slice)	90	
Fresh fruit in season – (apple, peach, etc)	70	
Hot or iced tea	10	345 Cal
SNACK		
Handful unsalted mixed nuts	100	
Coffee or tea	10	110 Cal
DINNER		
Healthy Chicken Salad (Day 69 Recipe - page 175)	330	
Small whole-grain roll	80	
Glass of white wine (4 oz)	100	
Water with lemon wedge	10	520 Cal
SNACK		
Kashi TLC Chewy Granola Bar	140	
Coffee or tea	10	150 Cal
		1505 Cal

84

Day 70 1500 Calorie Meal Plan

BREAKFAST	Calories	Totals
Orange juice (½ cup)	50	
Wild blueberry pancakes (Day 10 Recipe - page 116)	190	
Turkey bacon (2 slices)	70	
Light syrup (1½ Tbsp)	45	
Coffee	10	365 Cal
SNACK		
Yogurt (6 oz, nonfat, any flavor)	90	
Coffee or tea	10	100 Cal
LUNCH		
Peanut butter (2 Tbsp) on 2 slices of whole-grain bread	340	
Skim milk (6 oz)	65	
Unsweetened apple sauce (½ cup)	45	450 Cal
SNACK		
Fresh fruit in season (pear, peach, etc)	70	
Coffee or tea	10	80 Cal
DINNER		
Baked Cod (Day 70 Recipe - page 176)	230	
Brown rice (½ cup after cooking)	100	
Green beans - steamed	25	
Zucchini, tomatoes & onion – steamed	45	
Water	0	400 Cal
SNACK		
100-Calorie Pack Cookies	100	
Coffee or tea	10	110 Cal
		1505 Cal

Day 71 1500 Calorie Meal Plan

BREAKFAST	Calories	Totals
Fresh sliced orange	75	
Cheerios (1 cup) + ½ cup skim milk + about 15	190	
Whole grain toast (1 slice)	70	
Coffee	10	345 Cal
SNACK		
Handful unsalted mixed nuts	100	
Coffee or tea	10	110 Cal
LUNCH		
Cottage cheese (1 cup low fat)	180	
Large tossed salad with 1½ Tbsp low-cal dressing	70	
Small whole-grain roll	80	
Hot or iced tea	10	340 Cal
SNACK		
Fresh fruit in season (peach, plum, etc)	70	
Coffee or tea	10	80 Cal
DINNER		
Chicken Scaloppini (Day 71 Recipe - page 177)	260	
White Rice (½ cup – after cooking)	100	
Snow peas or green beans - steamed	25	
Whole-grain bread (1 slice)	70	
Water with lemon wedge	10	465 Cal
SNACK		
Blueberry muffin	145	
Coffee or tea	10	155 Cal
		1495 Cal

Day 72 1500 Calorie Meal Plan

BREAKFAST	Calories	Totals
Grapefruit (½)	75	
Scrambled egg	80	
Turkey bacon (2 slices)	70	
Whole-grain toast (1 slice)	70	
Coffee	10	305 Cal
SNACK		
Yogurt (6 oz, nonfat, any flavor)	90	
Coffee or tea	10	100 Cal
LUNCH		
Soup (Appendix B - page 202)	160	
Whole-grain bread (1 slice)	70	
Fresh fruit in season (peach, plum, etc)	70	
Water	0	300 Cal
SNACK		
Handful unsalted mixed nuts	100	
Coffee or tea	10	110 Cal
DINNER		
Eat Out – Fish dinner (Day 72 Recipe - page 178)		
Maximum allowable calories	595	595 Cal
SNACK		
Graham crackers (3 squares)	90	
Coffee or tea	10	100 Cal
		1510 Cal

Day 73 1500 Calorie Meal Plan

BREAKFAST	Calories	Totals
Orange juice (½ cup)	50	
Shredded Wheat (1 cup) + ½ cup skim milk + ½ banana	260	
Coffee	10	320 Cal
SNACK		
Fresh fruit in season (apple, plum, etc)	70	
Coffee or tea	10	80 Cal
LUNCH		
Turkey frank (2 oz) with mustard & relish	150	
Hot-dog bun	130	
Diet soda	0	280 Cal
SNACK		
Yogurt (6 oz, nonfat, any flavor)	90	
Coffee or tea	10	100 Cal
DINNER		
Pasta Pomodoro (Day 73 Recipe - page 179)	420	
Large tossed salad with 1½ Tbsp low-cal dressing	70	
Italian or French bread (1 slice)	80	
Water	0	570 Cal
SNACK		
Blueberry muffin (Day 42 Recipe - page 148)	145	
Coffee or tea	10	155 Cal
		1505 Cal

Day 74 1500 Calorie Meal Plan

BREAKFAST	Calories	Totals
Cantaloupe (½ medium)	50	
Wheaties (¾ cup) + ½ cup skim milk + ½ banana	190	
Blueberry Muffin	145	
Coffee	10	395 Cal
SNACK		
Fresh fruit in season (pear, plum, etc)	70	
Coffee or tea	10	80 Cal
LUNCH		
Grilled Swiss cheese sandwich (2 oz low-fat cheese)	320	
Pickle spear	0	
Hot or iced tea	10	330 Cal
SNACK		
Handful unsalted mixed nuts	100	
Coffee or tea	10	110 Cal
DINNER		
Frozen chicken dinner (Day 74 Recipe - page 180)	300	
Large tossed salad with 1½ Tbsp low-cal dressing	70	
Water with lemon wedge	10	380 Cal
SNACK		
Graham crackers (4 squares)	120	
Skim milk (6 oz)	70	190 Cal
		1485 Cal

Day 75 1500 Calorie Meal Plan

BREAKFAST	Calories	Totals
Grapefruit (½ medium)	50	
Smoothie (Day 14 Recipe - page 120)	220	
Coffee	10	280 Cal
SNACK		
Popcorn Mini Bag	110	
Coffee or tea	10	120 Cal
LUNCH		
Subway 6" (Roast Beef, Cheese + veggies)	245	
Hot or iced tea	10	255 Cal
SNACK		
Yogurt (6 oz, nonfat, any flavor)	90	
Coffee or tea	10	100 Cal
DINNER		
Szechuan Noodles & Pork (Day 75 Recipe - page 181)	440	
Large tossed salad with 1½ Tbsp low-cal dressing	70	
Fresh fruit in season (apple, peach, etc)	70	
Water with lemon wedge	10	590 Cal
SNACK		
Kashi TLC Chewy Granola Bar	140	
Coffee or tea	10	150 Cal
		1495 Cal

Day 76 1500 Calorie Meal Plan

BREAKFAST	Calories	Totals
Orange juice (½ cup)	50	
Kashi GoLean (1 cup) + ½ cup skim milk + ½ banana	235	
Coffee	10	295 Cal
SNACK		
Fresh fruit in season (apple, peach, etc)	70	
Coffee or tea	10	80 Cal
LUNCH		
Subway 6" (Ham, Cheese + veggies)	260	
Hot or iced tea	10	270 Cal
SNACK		
Popcorn Mini Bag	110	
Coffee or tea	10	120 Cal
DINNER		
Grilled Sea Scallops (Day 76 Recipe - page 182)	200	
Corn on the cob – one ear	100	
Tomato slices drizzled with Evoo	60	
Large tossed salad with 1½ Tbsp low-cal dressing	70	
Small whole-grain roll	80	
Glass red wine (4 oz)	100	
Water	0	610 Cal
SNACK		
Skinny Cow Low Fat Fudge Bar	100	100 Cal
		1485 Cal

Day 77 1500 Calorie Meal Plan

BREAKFAST	Calories	Totals
Orange juice (½ cup)	50	
Fried egg	80	
Turkey bacon (2 slices)	70	
Toasted raisin bread (1 slice)	75	
Coffee	10	285 Cal
SNACK		
Yogurt (6 oz, nonfat, any flavor)	90	
Coffee or tea	10	100 Cal
LUNCH		
Soup (Appendix B - page 202)	150	
Lettuce & tomato sandwich (Tbsp light mayo)	180	
Cucumber slices and carrots and celery sticks	15	
Hot or iced tea	10	355 Cal
SNACK		
Handful unsalted mixed nuts	100	
Coffee or tea	10	110 Cal
DINNER		
Chicken with Peppers & Rice (Day 77 Recipe - page 183)	290	
Large tossed salad with 1½ Tbsp low-cal dressing	70	
Whole-grain bread (1 slice)	70	
Fresh fruit in season (apple, peach, etc)	70	
Water	0	500 Cal
SNACK		
Dark chocolate (1 oz)	150	150 Cal
		1500 Cal

Day 78 1500 Calorie Meal Plan

BREAKFAST	Calories	Totals
Grapefruit (½)	75	
Cheerios (1 cup) + ½ cup skim milk + about 15 raisins	190	
Coffee	10	275 Cal
SNACK		
Fresh fruit in season (peach, plum, etc)	70	
Coffee or tea	10	80 Cal
LUNCH		
Cottage cheese (1 cup low fat)	180	
Large tossed salad with 1½ Tbsp low-cal dressing	70	
Small whole-grain roll	80	
Hot or iced tea	10	340 Cal
SNACK		
Handful unsalted mixed nuts	100	
Coffee or tea	10	110 Cal
DINNER		
Trout w Lemon Capers (Day 78 Recipe - page 184)	340	
Wild rice (½ cup – after cooking)	100	
Green beans (steamed)	30	
Sautéed cherry tomatoes (See page 131)	60	
Water with lemon wedge	10	540 Cal
SNACK		
Blueberry muffin	145	
Coffee or tea	10	155 Cal
		1500 Cal

Day 79 1500 Calorie Meal Plan

BREAKFAST	Calories	Totals
Grapefruit (½)	75	
Scrambled egg	80	
Whole-grain toast (1 slice)	70	
Coffee	10	235 Cal
SNACK		
Yogurt (6 oz, nonfat, any flavor)	90	
Coffee or tea	10	100 Cal
LUNCH		
Chorizo, Egg & Cheese*	260	
Diet soda or water	0	260 Cal
* Hot Pockets (wrap)		
SNACK		
Fresh fruit in season (apple, pear, etc)	70	
Coffee or tea	10	80 Cal
DINNER		
Eat Out – Chinese food (Day 79 Recipe - page 185)		
Max allowable calories	640	640 Cal
SNACK		
Graham crackers (4 squares)	120	
Skim milk (6 oz)	65	185 Cal
		1500 Cal

Day 80 1500 Calorie Meal Plan

BREAKFAST	Calories	Totals
Tomato juice (½ cup)	20	
Shredded Wheat (1 cup) + ½ cup skim milk + ½ banana	260	
Coffee	10	290 Cal
SNACK		
Handful unsalted mixed nuts	100	
Coffee or tea	10	110 Cal
LUNCH		
Left over Chinese food from Day 79	260	
Water	0	270 Cal
SNACK		
Yogurt (6 oz, nonfat, any flavor)	90	
Coffee or tea	10	100 Cal
DINNER		
Vegetable Chili (Day 80 Recipe - page 186)	360	
Brown rice (½ cup – after cooking)	100	
Large tossed salad with 1½ Tbsp low-cal dressing	70	
Whole-grain bread (1 slice)	70	
Water	0	600 Cal
SNACK		
Kashi TLC Chewy Granola Bar	140	140 Cal
		1510 Cal

Day 81 1500 Calorie Meal Plan

BREAKFAST	Calories	Totals
Cantaloupe (½ medium)	50	
Oatmeal (½ cup dry) + ½ cup skim milk + about 15 raisins	220	
Coffee	10	280 Cal
SNACK		
Handful unsalted mixed nuts	100	
Coffee or tea	10	110 Cal
LUNCH		
Turkey breast (2 oz) sandwich	245	
Lettuce, tomato and Tbsp light mayo	35	
Pickle spear	0	
Fresh fruit in season (peach, pear, etc)	70	
Water	0	350 Cal
SNACK		
Dark chocolate (1 oz)	150	
Coffee or tea	10	160 Cal
DINNER		
Frozen meat dinner (Day 81 Recipe - page 187)	300	
Large tossed salad with 1½ Tbsp low-cal dressing	70	
Whole-grain bread (1 slice)	70	
Water with lemon wedge	10	450 Cal
SNACK		
Graham crackers (3 squares)	90	
Skim milk (6 oz)	65	155 Cal
		1505 Cal

Day 82 1500 Calorie Meal Plan

BREAKFAST	Calories	Totals
Fresh or frozen strawberries (1 cup)	25	
French toasted English Muffin (Day 3 Recipe - page 109)	270	
Light syrup (1 Tbsp)	30	
Coffee	10	335 Cal
SNACK		
Fresh fruit in season (apple, peach, etc)	70	
Coffee or tea	10	80 Cal
LUNCH		
Subway 6" (Roast Beef, Cheese + veggies)*	245	
Canned pineapple (1 cup, no-sugar-added juice)	80	
Hot or iced tea	10	335 Cal
SNACK		
Popcorn Mini Bag	110	110 Cal
DINNER		
Chinese Chicken Salad (Day 82 Recipe - page 188)	440	
Hot or iced tea	10	450 Cal
SNACK		
Blueberry muffin	145	
Skim milk (4 oz)	45	190 Cal
		1505 Cal

Day 83 1500 Calorie Meal Plan

BREAKFAST	Calories	Totals
Orange juice (½ cup)	50	
Wheaties (¾ cup) + ½ cup skim milk + ½ banana	190	
Whole-grain toast (1 slice)	70	
Coffee	10	320 Cal
SNACK		
Handful unsalted mixed nuts	100	
Coffee or tea	10	110 Cal
LUNCH		
Ham (2 oz) with mustard on 2 slices rye bread	300	
Pickle spear	0	
Small bunch of grapes	65	
Hot or iced tea	10	375 Cal
SNACK		
Yogurt (6 oz, nonfat, any flavor)	90	
Coffee or tea	10	100 Cal
DINNER		
Lentil Soup (Day 83 Recipe - page 189)	260	
Large tossed salad with 1½ Tbsp low-cal dressing	70	
Small whole-grain roll	80	
Fresh fruit in season (apple, peach, etc)	70	
Water with lemon wedge	10	490 Cal
SNACK		
100-Calorie Pack Cookies	100	
Coffee or tea	10	110 Cal
		1505 Cal

Day 84 1500 Calorie Meal Plan

BREAKFAST	Calories	Totals
Fresh orange sliced	75	
Soft-boiled egg	80	
Whole grain toast (2 slices)	140	
Coffee	10	305 Cal
SNACK		
Yogurt (6 oz, nonfat, any flavor)	90	
Coffee or tea	10	100 Cal
LUNCH		
Salad – 3 oz canned salmon, 1 tsp Evoo, onions & celery	200	
Lettuce & tomato wedges	20	
Rye bread (1 slice)	70	
Fresh fruit in season (apple, plum, etc)	70	
Coffee or tea	10	370 Cal
SNACK		
Handful unsalted mixed nuts	100	
Coffee or tea	10	110 Cal
DINNER		
Turkey Burger (Day 84 Recipe - page 190)	360	
Green beans or asparagus - steamed	25	
Pickle spear	0	
Large tossed salad with 1½ Tbsp low-cal dressing	70	
Water with lemon wedge	10	465 Cal
SNACK		
Blueberry muffin	145	
Coffee or tea	10	155 Cal
		1505 Cal

Day 85 1500 Calorie Meal Plan

BREAKFAST	Calories	Totals
Grapefruit (½)	75	
Cheerios (1 cup) + ½ cup skim milk + about 15 raisins	190	
Coffee	10	275 Cal
SNACK		
Fresh fruit in season (apple, peach, etc)	70	
Coffee or tea	10	80 Cal
LUNCH		
Cottage cheese (1 cup low fat)	180	
Large tossed salad with 1½ Tbsp low-cal dressing	70	
Small whole-grain roll	80	
Hot or iced tea	10	340 Cal
SNACK		
Handful unsalted mixed nuts	100	
Coffee or tea	10	110 Cal
DINNER		
Meat Loaf (Day 85 Recipe - page 191)	290	
One-half acorn squash (baked with ½ tsp maple	90	
Spinach (½ cup steamed & drizzled with 1 tsp	70	
Whole-grain bread (1 slice)	70	
Gelatin dessert (unsweetened)	10	
Water with lemon wedge	10	540 Cal
SNACK		
Kashi TLC Chewy Granola Bar	140	
Coffee or tea	10	150 Cal
		1495 Cal

Day 86 1500 Calorie Meal Plan

BREAKFAST	Calories	Totals
Cantaloupe (½ medium)	50	
Fried eggs (2 eggs)	160	
Toasted whole-grain bread (2 slices)	140	
Coffee	10	360 Cal
SNACK		
Yogurt (6 oz, nonfat, any flavor)	90	
Coffee or tea	10	100 Cal
LUNCH		
Soup (Appendix B - page 202)	200	
Hard whole-grain roll (medium)	80	
Lettuce & tomato slices	20	
Hot or iced tea	10	310 Cal
SNACK		
Carrot sticks + ¼ cup low-fat cottage cheese & chives	60	
Coffee or tea	10	70 Cal
DINNER		
Tuna & Bean Salad (Day 86 Recipe - page 192)	355	
Small whole-grain roll	80	
Fresh fruit in season (apple, plum, etc)	70	
Water	0	505 Cal
SNACK		
Blueberry muffin	145	
Coffee or tea	10	155 Cal
		1500 Cal

Day 87 1500 Calorie Meal Plan

BREAKFAST	Calories	Totals
Cantaloupe (½ medium)	50	
Smoothie (Day 14 Recipe - page 120)	220	
Coffee	10	280 Cal
SNACK		
Fresh fruit in season (peach, plum, etc)	70	
Coffee or tea	10	80 Cal
LUNCH		
Leftover meat loaf (½ of Day 85 serving)	145	
Whole-grain bread (1 slice)	70	
Lettuce & tomato slices	20	
Hot or iced tea	10	245 Cal
SNACK		
Handful unsalted mixed nuts	100	
Coffee or tea	10	110 Cal
DINNER		
Pasta Primavera (Day 87 Recipe - page 193)	460	
Large tossed salad with 1½ Tbsp low-cal dressing	70	
Italian or French bread (1 slice)	80	
Water with lemon wedge	10	620 Cal
SNACK		
Skinny Cow Ice Cream Sandwich	140	
Coffee or tea	10	150 Cal
		1485 Cal

Day 88 1500 Calorie Meal Plan

BREAKFAST	Calories	Totals
Tomato juice (½ cup)	20	
Shredded Wheat (1 cup) + ½ cup skim milk + ½ banana	260	
Coffee	10	290 Cal
SNACK		
Handful unsalted mixed nuts	100	
Coffee or tea	10	110 Cal
LUNCH		
Subway 6" (Ham, Cheese + veggies)	260	
Fresh fruit in season (apple, peach, etc)	70	
Hot or iced tea	10	340 Cal
SNACK		
Kashi TLC Chewy Granola Bar	140	
Coffee or tea	10	150 Cal
DINNER		
Frozen chicken dinner (Day 88 Recipe - page 194)	300	
Large tossed salad with 1½ Tbsp low-cal dressing	70	
Whole-grain bread (1 slice)	70	
Water	0	440 Cal
SNACK		
Graham crackers (4 squares)	120	
Skim milk (4 oz)	45	165 Cal
		1495 Cal

Day 89 1500 Calorie Meal Plan

BREAKFAST	Calories	Totals
Orange juice (½ cup)	50	
Wild blueberry pancakes (Day 10 Recipe - page 116)	190	
Turkey bacon (2 slices)	70	
Light syrup (1½ Tbsp)	45	
Coffee	10	365 Cal
SNACK		
Yogurt (6 oz, nonfat, any flavor)	90	
Coffee or tea	10	100 Cal
LUNCH		
Salad (3 oz canned tuna, 1 tsp Evoo, onions, celery)	175	
Lettuce & tomato wedges	20	
Rye bread (1 slice)	70	
Fresh fruit in season (apple, peach, etc)	70	
Water	0	335 Cal
SNACK		
Handful unsalted mixed nuts	100	
Coffee or tea	10	110 Cal
DINNER		
Fish stew (Day 89 Recipe - page 195)	300	
Large tossed salad with 1½ Tbsp low-cal dressing	70	
Whole-grain bread (1 slice)	70	
Water	0	440 Cal
SNACK		
Kashi TLC Chewy Granola Bar	140	
Coffee or tea	10	150 Cal
		1500 Cal

Day 90 1500 Calorie Meal Plan

BREAKFAST	Calories	Totals
Fresh orange sliced	75	
Kashi GoLean (1 cup) + ½ cup skim milk + ½ banana	235	
Coffee	10	320 Cal
SNACK		
Fresh fruit in season (pear, plum, etc)	70	
Coffee or tea	10	80 Cal
LUNCH		
Soup (Appendix B - page 202)	130	
Large tossed salad with 1½ Tbsp low-cal dressing	70	
Whole-grain bread (1 slice)	70	
Hot or iced tea	10	280 Cal
SNACK		
Graham crackers (3 squares)	90	
Coffee or tea	10	100 Cal
DINNER		
Veal w Mushrooms & Tomato -Day 90 Recipe - page 196	520	
Small whole-grain roll	80	
Water with lemon wedge	10	610 Cal
SNACK		
Popcorn Mini Bag	110	
Coffee or tea	10	120 Cal
		1510 Cal

Recipes and Diet Tips

Day 1- Recipe

Chicken with Peppers & Onions

4 boneless and skinless chicken breasts (about 5 oz each)
Coat the chicken breasts in a bottled barbeque sauce. Prepare medium-hot fire on well-oiled grill. Place breasts on grill, turning them every 4 minutes, for 10 to 12 minutes, or until done. (To check if breasts are done, the meat should be moist and white with no sign of pink when you cut into the breast.) Salt and pepper to taste.
2 medium red peppers, sliced
1 medium onion, sliced
Place peppers and onions in pan with 2 tablespoons fat-free chicken stock. Sauté until stock is reduced. Spray pan lightly with non-stick cooking oil and cook another 2 minutes. Salt and pepper to taste.
Serves 4. About 250 Calories per serving (for chicken only).

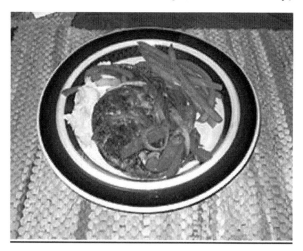

Diet Tip of the Day: Weight Loss – take it one step, one meal, one workout, one day at a time. Just think of where you'll be in 90 days!

Day 2 - Recipe

Baked Herb-Crusted Cod

4 cod fish fillets (4 to 5 ounces each)
2 tablespoons flour
2 tablespoons cornmeal
2 tablespoons minced fresh herbs
2 teaspoons lemon juice

Sprinkle cod with lemon juice. Mix flour, cornmeal and herbs and dust the cod with the cornmeal-herb mixture. Bake in oven at 375 °F for 10 minutes. Add salt and black pepper to taste.

Serves 4. One serving is about 230 Calories (for cod only).

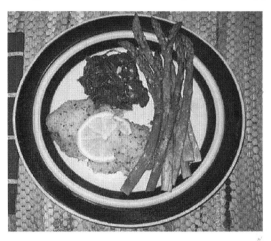

Diet Tip of the Day:. A **reducing diet is best supervised by a physician**. This is especially true when a great deal of weight needs to be lost, or if you have an ailment or a history of medical problems.

Day 3 - Recipe

French-Toasted English Muffin

6 whole wheat light English muffins, sliced in half
4 eggs
2 cups skim milk
2 teaspoons vanilla
A dash of cinnamon
In a medium bowl, beat together eggs and skim milk. Add vanilla and cinnamon. Slice English muffins into halves and saturate slices in egg mixture. In a non-stick skillet coated with cooking spray, cook muffins until both sides are golden brown. Dust lightly with confectionary sugar. Serve hot or keep in an oven or warmer at 200 °F until ready to plate. **Serves 4**. Three English muffin slices per serving. Serving is 270 Calories.

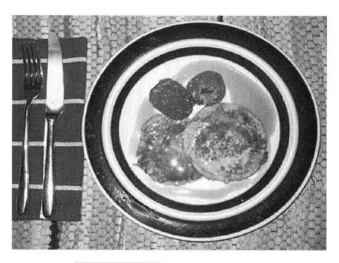

Diet Tip of the Day: **"Eat Slowly"** This is especially vital when you are trying to lose weight. If you are someone who eats fast, who finishes before everyone else at the table, you are not giving yourself a chance to feel full. While everyone else is still eating, you either sit there and pick, or you have seconds, taking in extra calories you could avoid if you would just slow down.

Day 4 - Recipe

Carrie's Low-Cal Meat Loaf

½ pound ground white meat turkey
½ pound ground beef (about 90% lean)
1 large egg
½ cup skim milk
¼ cup bread crumbs
¼ cup ketchup
¼ cup chopped carrots
¼ cup chopped onion

In a medium bowl, combine all ingredients. Add salt and pepper to taste. Mix until blended and form into a loaf. Place loaf into oven preheated to 350 °F. Bake until an instant-read thermometer inserted in the center of the loaf reads 160 °F. This should take about one hour.

Shown below is meat loaf, acorn squash (baked with 1 teaspoon of maple syrup). Also shown is steamed spinach drizzled with extra-virgin olive oil. **Serves 5**. About 290 Calories per serving (for meat loaf only). Note: reserve half a serving of the meat loaf which is to be eaten for lunch on Day 6.

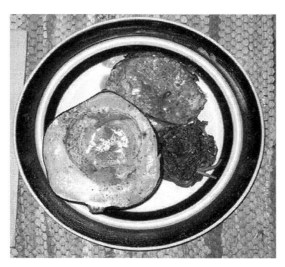

Diet Tip of the Day: **Take a daily multi-vitamin/mineral supplement.** This is very important when you're on a diet – as a kind of insurance policy.

Day 5 - Recipe

Frozen-Fish Dinner

No recipe today. No cooking today. It's your day off! Some reasonably good frozen fish dinners are:

Seafood	Shrimp Alfredo	Lean Cuisine	~~230~~ 240
Seafood	Tuna Noodle Casserole	Smart Ones	~~250~~ 270
Seafood	Shrimp & Angel Hair Pasta	Lean Cuisine	~~280~~ 290
Seafood	Parmesan Crusted Fish	Lean Cuisine	~~290~~ 300
Seafood	Tortilla Crusted Fish	Lean Cuisine	~~300~~ 310

That's it. At this writing, there are just not that many frozen fish dinners for sale at supermarkets, although new entrees are being introduced continually. If you choose any of the above entrees, you will not use all of the **340 Calories allocated for this meal**. In this case, use the excess calories anyway you wish. Splurge on extra dessert or save the calories for another day!

See **Appendix A** on page 197 for our comprehensive list of frozen entrees. Please read the important **Frozen-Food Safety Warning** in **Appendix C** on page 203.

Diet Tip of the Day: **Buy a pedometer** and start walking. For the average person 2100 steps amounts to walking about one mile. A Harvard study has shown that 8000 to 10,000 step per day promote weight loss. And you're not obliged to walk continuously until you accrue all 10,000 steps. Rather, all steps throughout the day to wherever and whenever count toward your daily total. Because 10,000 steps a day may not be achievable by some people, particularly those who are elderly, sedentary, or who have chronic diseases, rather than insisting on a blanket 10,000 steps per day, your initial stepping goal should your baseline steps plus an increment of an additional 2500 steps . (Your baseline being the number of steps you take in an average day.)

Day 6 - Recipe

Grandma's Pizza

The following is a pizza recipe used by Gail Johnson's Italian grandmother. She was from a small mountain village located between Rome and Naples.

Pizza dough: To save time use prepared dough, preferably whole wheat. To start, flour a large cutting board. Divide one pound of prepared pizza dough into four parts. Roll out each dough ball as thin as possible.

Tomato sauce: Sauté ½ small onion, chopped fine, in 1 teaspoon olive oil. Add two finely chopped garlic cloves, 1½ cups chopped plum tomatoes and ½ teaspoon chopped fresh oregano. Stir and cook about 5 minutes on a low flame.

Pizza preparation & cooking: On each pizza, spread evenly ¼ cup of the tomato sauce. Add ½ ounce of shredded part-skim mozzarella cheese, 1 teaspoon Parmesan cheese, 3 slices of a Portobello mushroom, some torn fresh basil, and drizzle with extra-virgin olive oil. Put pizzas on a pan and place in 475 °F oven for about 15 to 20 minutes, or until crust is crisp and cheese is just melting. (Freeze left over sauce for use on Day 13.)

<u>Serves 4</u>. Each pizza contains approximately 350 Calories.

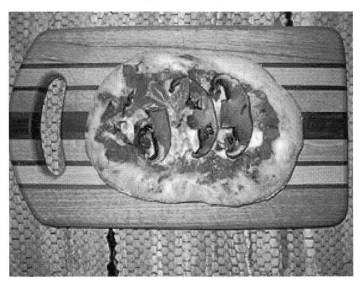

<u>Diet Tip of the Day:</u> For **life-long weight control** take a vigorous 30 to 60 minute walk everyday! That's right – everyday. Make exercise a nonflexible top priority part of your life. When it comes to exercise the key words are consistent, persistent, unyielding, dogged. Get the point?

Day 7 - Recipe

<u>Chicken Dinner - Out</u>

No recipe today. No cooking today. Have a chicken dinner at your favorite restaurant, but make sure you choose a restaurant where you have a fighting chance to achieve your calorie goal. For your chicken dinner out, your maximum allowable calories (includes appetizer, soup, main course and dessert) are as follows:

- For the **1200 Calorie Diet**: 530 Calories
- For the **1500 Calorie Diet**: 630 Calories
- For the **1800 Calorie Diet**: 630 Calories

Tips for Eating Chicken Out: First, order simple and order skinless white meat only, such as broiled chicken breast with steamed vegetables and brown rice. Tell the waiter you want no sauce, no gravy, nothing added. Then, knowing your calorie objective, and that chicken is about 50 Calories per ounce, most steamed vegetable servings average approximately 50 Calories per cup, and rice is about 100 Calories per ½ cup, decide how much to eat – and take the remainder home. If fresh fruit is not an option, pass on dessert and have the evening snack specified for that day in this diet.

In a restaurant, most nutritionists recommend you eat the low-calorie items on your plate first. Start with the salad, soup and veggies. By the time you get to the chicken and starches you will hopefully be full enough to be content with smaller portions of the higher-calorie choices. (Incidentally, feel free to substitute skinless white meat turkey for chicken.)

Finally, some dieticians advise their dieting clients not to eat out. That's right. They believe eating at home is safer. But our thought is you have to eat out eventually so why not learn how while your resolve is high?

<u>Diet Tip of the Day:</u> When you're on a diet, eating in a restaurant can be a challenge, because most restaurant portions are huge, and can easily total more than 1000 Calories. So, in a restaurant decide how much to eat – and take the remainder home. A good general rule of thumb is to **eat half and bring the rest home**.

Day 8 - Recipe

<u>Baked Salmon with Salsa</u>

This is a simple, straight-forward recipe. The advantage of a simple recipe is there are no hidden calories.

4   5 oz salmon fillets
6   tablespoons bottled tomato-pepper salsa

Brown salmon fillets in non-stick pan and then place them in a baking dish. Cook fillets in an oven preheated to 350 °F for about 10 minutes. Plate the salmon. Stir bottled tomato-pepper salsa and spoon it over the salmon. <u>**Serves 4**</u>. One salmon fillet is about 215 Calories.

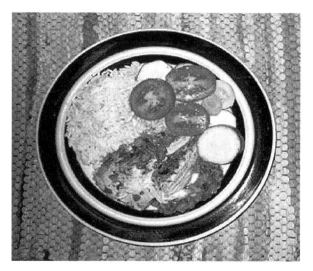

<u>**Diet Tip of the Day:**</u> Hunger is your body's way of telling you that you need calories. But **when you're done eating, you should feel better – satisfied but not stuffed**.

Day 9 - Recipe

Veggie Burger

Vegetable-based burgers can be purchased at your local supermarket. Patties of a veggie burger are made from either vegetables, soy, nuts, mushrooms, textured vegetable protein, dairy, or a combination of these foods.

In the U.S., two popular veggie burgers are the Boca Burger and Gardenburger. The Boca Burger is made chiefly from soy protein and wheat gluten. (Boca Burger patties are 2.5 oz each and range from 60 to 90 Calories.) The original Gardenburger is made from mushrooms, onions, brown rice, rolled oats, cheese, and spices. (Gardenburger patties are 2.5 oz each and about 100 Calories.)

To prepare, follow package directions. The version shown below has an added slice of low-fat cheddar cheese. The lettuce, tomato and ketchup shown actually add very few extra calories.

The veggie burger patty plus low-fat cheese amounts to approximately 150 Calories. Add a seeded roll and the total rises to 290 Calories.

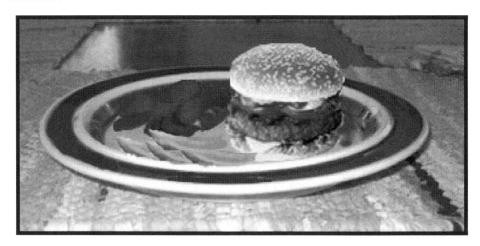

Diet Tip of the Day: **Drink lots of water** – about 8 glasses per day when you're trying to lose weight. Add a slice of lemon to make it more interesting. Often, when you think you're hungry, you are just thirsty. So, next time you crave a snack, drink some water first and see if that does it for you.

Day 10 - Recipe

Wild Blueberry Pancakes

This recipe makes a relatively low calorie, wholesome batch of delicious wild blueberry-whole wheat-buttermilk pancakes.

1 cup whole-wheat flour
1 cup buttermilk
1 egg
1 tablespoon vegetable oil
1 teaspoon baking powder
½ teaspoon baking soda

Stir ingredients until blended. Add ¾ cup fresh of frozen blueberries and gently stir. Using medium heat, preheat a non-stick skillet coated with cooking spray. Pour slightly less than ¼ cup of batter onto skillet per pancake. Cook slowly until bubbles break on surface of pancake. Turn and cook until other side is lightly browned.

Makes 8 pancakes. Pictured below are wild-blueberry pancakes with two slices of turkey bacon.
Serves 4. Each pancake is about 95 Calories

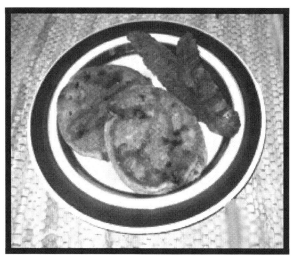

Bacon allowable only on 1500 and 1800 Calorie diets.

Diet Tip of the Day: Most experts associate eating a substantial breakfast with successful weight loss.

Day 11 - Recipe

Artichoke-Bean Salad

19-ounce can white kidney beans
10 artichoke hearts, quartered
⅓ cup chopped oregano
⅓ cup chopped parsley
3 cloves garlic, chopped
1 lemon, juiced
Combine ingredients in medium-size bowl. Stir in ¼ cup extra-virgin olive oil. Salt and black pepper to taste.
Serves 6. Approximately 190 Calories per serving.

Pictured on the plate below is the artichoke-bean salad as a side dish with two grilled chicken sausage links, tomato salsa and steamed green beans. Incidentally, this artichoke-bean combination over mixed salad greens served with a whole-grain bread makes a delicious, nutritious and reasonable low-calorie main course.

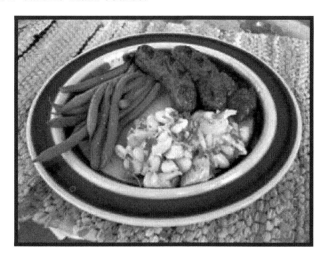

Diet Tip of the Day: Before you go to a **party**, have a small meal, such as a hardboiled egg, an apple, and a thirst quencher (like water, tea, seltzer, or diet soda). This will take the edge off your appetite and make it easier to resist the high-calorie goodies.

Day 12 - Recipe

Fish Dinner - Out

No recipe today. No cooking today. Have a fish dinner at your favorite restaurant, but make sure you choose a restaurant where you have a good chance to achieve your calorie goal. For today, your **goal for dinner is a maximum of 595 Calories**. This includes appetizer, soup, main course and dessert.

Tips for Eating Fish Out: The following is almost an exact repeat of the advice given eating out on previous days. First, order simple, such as broiled fish with steamed vegetables and brown rice. Tell the waiter you want no sauce, no gravy, nothing added. Then, knowing your calorie objective, and that fish is about 50 Calories per ounce, most steamed vegetable servings average approximately 50 Calories per cup, and rice is about 100 Calories per ½ cup, decide how much to eat – and take the remainder home. If fresh fruit is not an option, pass on dessert and have the evening snack specified for that day in the diet.

In a restaurant, some nutritionists recommend you eat the low-calorie items on your plate first. Start with the salad, soup and veggies. By the time you get to the fish and starches you will hopefully be full enough to be content with smaller portions of the higher-calorie choices.

Diet Tip of the Day: Phytonutrients are found in plant foods such as fruits, vegetables, whole grains, dried beans, nuts and seeds. Unlike protein, fat, vitamins and minerals, phytonutrients are not necessary for life, but evidence is growing that phytonutrients have many beneficial qualities.

Day 13 - Recipe

Pasta with Marinara Sauce

Prepare the sauce as you did for the Day 6 pizza (on page 112). But because the pizza sauce is a bit too thick, we add ¼ cup of pasta liquid to thin it. (The spiral pasta profile shown below is called fusilli, a very popular pasta shape because all those ridges hold buckets of tomato sauce.)
½ pound whole-wheat pasta
¼ teaspoon salt
Prepare the marinara tomato sauce as per Day 6 sauce but dilute it with ¼ cup of today's pasta liquid.

Bring 2 quarts of lightly salted water to a boil. Add pasta and stir occasionally (to keep pasta from sticking to the bottom of the pot). Keep water boiling and cook until pasta are "al dente." (Cooking time is approximately 9 minutes.) Drain pasta, add marinara sauce and serve hot. **Serves 4.** One serving is about 225 Calories.

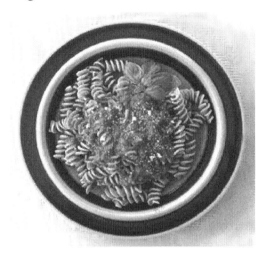

Diet Tip of the Day: **Beware of alcoholic beverages**. Beer has about 13 Calories per ounce, wine 25 Calories per ounce and whiskey a whopping 71 Calories per ounce.

Day 14 - Recipe
Low-Cal Smoothie

Smoothies are delicious, nutritious and fun to drink! They're great for a fast but nutritious breakfast, a light energy-boosting lunch, a healthy snack, a late afternoon pick me up, and a delicious dessert. Making your own smoothie is a smart way to save money and get healthy at the same time!

8 ounces plain fat-free yogurt
1 cup orange juice
1 cup strawberries
½ cup blueberries
1 banana
1 teaspoon sugar
1 teaspoon vanilla extract

Place yogurt, strawberries, and blueberries in a blender. Pour in orange juice. Add sugar and vanilla extract to mixture. Blend all ingredients until thick and smooth. Pour smoothie into a glass and enjoy.

Serves 2. About 220 Calories per serving

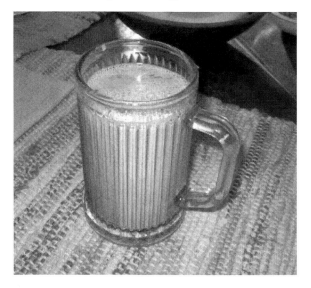

Diet Tip of the Day: Two scientific journals indicate **dark chocolate** - not white chocolate or milk chocolate - is potent antioxidant and is good for you. But don't overdo it, because you have to offset the extra chocolate calories by eating less of other foods.

Day 15 - Recipe

London Broil

1 lb boneless flank steak about ¾" thick, fat trimmed
1 clove garlic
1 teaspoon dry oregano
Rub each side of the flank steak with garlic. Season with oregano, salt and pepper to taste. Prepare a large non-stick skillet over high heat. Steak should sizzle when placed on hot skillet. Sear steak on one side for about 5 minutes; then turn and sear other side for about 4 minutes, or until done to preference. Check the center by making small incision. Carve into ¼-inch slices.
Serves 4. About 320 Calories per serving (for meat only).

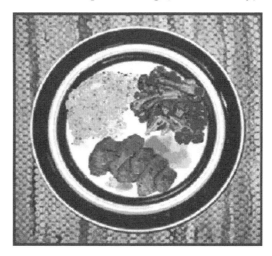

Diet Tip of the Day: Stay Busy. Most people will do anything to avoid work, housework, yard work, exercise, etc. But any kind of work burns a lot more calories than just sitting! Whatever it is you are avoiding – just go do it!

Day 16 - Recipe
Red Snapper with Special Sauce

    4   4-ounce red snapper fillets (salmon fillets okay)
    ½ cup white wine
    ½ cup non-fat yogurt mixed with ¼ cup mustard
    ½ pound green beans
    ¾ pint cherry tomatoes (about 20), halved
    4 teaspoons olive oil
    ¾ cup wild rice, brown rice and wheat berry mix.

Brown fillets in non-stick pan. Place fillets skin side down in baking dish coated with non-stick spray. Add white wine and cook in oven preheated to 350 ºF for about 15 minutes . Spoon pan juices over fillets. Salt and pepper to taste.

Place green beans in skillet. Add ¼-inch of water and cook over medium heat until water boils off. Add cherry tomatoes and olive oil. Stir well and sauté for a few minutes. (If desired, season with fresh rosemary and oregano.) Salt and pepper to taste.

Prepare rice mix per package directions.

Plate red snapper fillet and spoon over yogurt-mustard sauce. Add green beans and tomato mix and the wild rice mix. Serve hot.

Serves 4. One plate consisting of a snapper fillet (215 Cal) with green beans & tomato mix (75 Cal) and wild rice (160 Cal) totals 450 Calories.

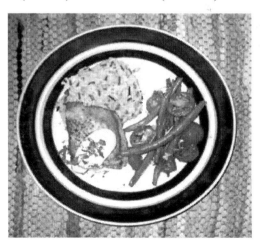

Diet Tip of the Day: **Don't have sweets in your house**. This makes them easier to resist. Out of sight, out of mind!

Day 17 - Recipe

Cajun Chicken Salad

This is a perfect after-work, quick, nutritious and delicious dinner.

4 boneless and skinless chicken breasts - about 5 oz each

4 teaspoons of bottled Cajun herb-spice mix

8 ounces mixed salad greens

¾ pint cherry tomatoes (about 20), halved

12 pitted black olives

2 tablespoons bottled light salad dressing

Brush chicken breasts lightly with olive oil. Roll breasts in Cajun herb-spice mix.

Brown breasts on non-stick oven-proof skillet. After breasts are brown, put skillet in 350 °F oven for approximately 15 minutes, or until done. (When the breasts are done, the meat should be moist and white with no sign of pink.) Cut breasts into ½-inch slices.

Serve hot or keep in an oven or warmer at 200 °F until ready to plate. Place chicken slices over a bed of mixed salad greens. Add tomatoes, olives and two tablespoons of your favorite low-calorie salad dressing. **Serves 4**. 330 Calories per serving

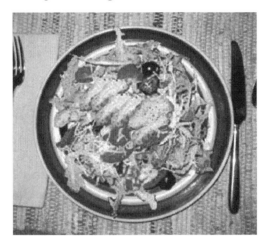

Diet Tip of the Day: Hot or cold cereal topped with fruit, and fat-free milk makes a nutritious, relatively low-calorie meal anytime.

Day 18 - Recipe

Grilled Swordfish

1¼ pounds swordfish
1 bottle citrus-herb marinade
¾ pint cherry tomatoes (about 20), halved
4 medium potatoes
2 cups fresh spinach
1 teaspoon rosemary & juice of ¼ lemon
2 teaspoon extra-virgin olive oil, divided
Steam spinach with garlic and drizzle with about 1 teaspoon extra-virgin olive oil.

Cut potatoes in medium-size pieces and sprinkle with lemon juice, add rosemary, salt and black pepper. Place potatoes on grill for about 10 minutes, turning occasionally.

Toss cherry tomatoes in remaining extra-virgin olive oil. Add fresh oregano, salt and black pepper. Place on heavy-duty aluminum foil, seal and grill for about 3 minutes.

Marinade swordfish in citrus-herb vinaigrette. Grill on hot fire for about 5 minutes on one side and 3 minutes on the other, or until done as desired. **Serves 4**. One plate of grilled swordfish (250 Calories) with potatoes (100 Calories), cherry tomatoes (45 Calories) and steamed spinach (50 Calories) totals 445 Calories.

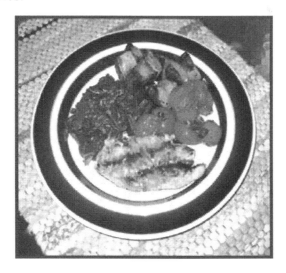

Day 19 - Recipe

Chinese Dinner - Out

No recipe today. No cooking today. Have a Chinese dinner at your favorite restaurant, but make sure you choose a restaurant where you have a reasonable chance to achieve your calorie goal. For today, **your goal for dinner is a maximum of 640 Calories**. This includes any appetizer, soup, main course and any dessert.

Tips for Eating Chinese: You can consume a lot of calories in a Chinese restaurant – if you order carelessly. For example a typical portion of General Tso's chicken is loaded with about 1000 Calories, then add another 200 Calories for a cup of rice.

First rule, order simple. Look for an entree with lots of vegetables, some fish or chicken and brown rice. Tell the waiter you want your food steamed with any sauce on the side. (This is not only a low-calorie way of eating Chinese food but is also the most nutritious way to eat Chinese food.)

Then, knowing your 640 Calorie objective, and that chicken and fish are about 50 Calories per ounce, most steamed vegetable servings average approximately 50 Calories per cup, and rice is about 200 Calories per cup, decide how much of the meal you can eat – and take the remainder home. (Note that you will be eating half a serving of left over Chinese food for lunch tomorrow.) To stay within your maximum allowable calorie total, you should pass on dessert and have the evening snack specified for that day in the diet.

Incidentally, although Chinese is specified, feel free to substitute Thai food, Vietnamese, Indian, Middle Eastern, or any other favorite ethnic food. Just make sure you don't exceed the maximum allowable 640 calories for this meal.

Diet Tip of the Day: Another dilemma for dieters is **judging portion size**. It makes no sense to worry about whether to apportion 70 or 80 Calories per ounce for a cut of lean meat if you have no idea whether the portion you are planning to eat weighs four or ten ounces. To be successful, you must learn to estimate portion sizes with reasonable accuracy.

Day 20 - Recipe

Quick Pasta alla Puttanesca

This famous pasta dish originated in Naples Italy. Puttanesca means "ladies of the night." Although the exact origin of the name is unclear, one thing is clear: It's delicious! Here is one of many recipe versions.

½ pound spaghetti (whole wheat preferred)
20 black or green pitted olives
14.5-oz can diced tomatoes
4 oz tomato sauce
2 tablespoon extra-virgin olive oil
3 cloves of garlic, chopped
1 tablespoon dried minced onion
½ teaspoon crushed red pepper flakes
1 tablespoon capers drained and rinsed
¼ cup currants

Cook spaghetti according to package directions. Drain and return spaghetti to pot; add a teaspoon extra-virgin olive oil and toss to coat.

Heat remaining olive oil in large skillet over medium-high heat. Add red pepper flakes; cook and stir 1 to 2 minutes or until sizzling. Add onion and garlic; cook and stir 1 minute. Add canned tomatoes with juice, tomato sauce, olives, currants and capers. Cook over medium-high heat, stirring frequently, until sauce is heated through.

Serves 4. About 345 Calories per serving

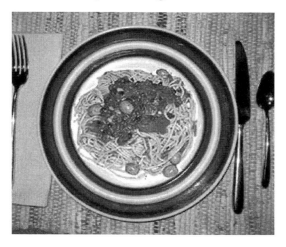

Diet Tip of the Day: Dilute fruit juices, such as apple juice, orange, etc. with water. This cuts the flavor slightly but really reduces calorie content.

Day 21 - Recipe

Frozen-Meat Dinner

No recipe today. No cooking today. Another day off! That's it. At this writing, there are just not that many frozen meat dinners for sale at supermarkets, although new entrees are being introduced continually. Here are some reasonably good frozen-meat dinners:

Meat	Steak Portobella	Lean Cuisine	160
Meat	Asian Style Beef & Broccoli	Smart Ones	~~160~~ 170
Meat	Beef Merlot	Healthy Choice	180
Meat	Home style Beef Pot Roast	Smart Ones	180
Meat	Salisbury Steak with Mac & Cheese	Lean Cuisine	~~270~~ 290
Pasta	Pasta with Swedish Meatballs	Smart Ones	~~280~~ 290
Meat	Classic Meat Loaf	Healthy Choice	300

If you choose most of the above entrees, you will fall well short of the **300 Calories allocated for this day**. In this case, use the remaining calories anyway you wish. Indulge on extra dessert or save the calories for another day.

See **Appendix A** on page 197 for our comprehensive list of frozen entrees. Please read the important **Frozen-Food Safety Warning** in **Appendix C** on page 203.

Diet Tip of the Day: Understanding nutrition is not only vital for good health but also will help you control your weight over the long term. For example, did you know that foods that are labeled an "excellent source" of a particular nutrient provide 20% or more of the Recommended Daily Value. Whereas, foods that are a "good source" of a nutrient provide between 10 and 20% of the Recommended Daily Value.

Day 22 - Recipe

Shrimp & Spinach Salad

2 pounds shrimp in shell
½ pound small green beans, trimmed
½ pound baby spinach leaves
2 tablespoon lemon juice
¼ cup extra-virgin olive oil
2 teaspoon minced fresh dill
1 tablespoon minced green onion

To make vinaigrette, combine lemon juice, olive oil, dill, salt and black pepper to taste and whisk until blended. Stir in minced onion and set aside. Steam green beans and set aside.

Peel, de-vein and butterfly shrimp. Place shrimp in a bowl and add water to cover. Add 1 teaspoon of salt, and let stand for 10 minutes. Drain, rinse, drain again, and dry. Arrange shrimp in broiling pan without a rack. Brush shrimp with a little of the vinaigrette and place under preheated broiler, about 3 inches from heat. Broil about 3 to 4 minutes, turning shrimp once, or until both sides turn pink.

Remove shrimp from broiler and add remaining vinaigrette and green beans to the broiling pan. Stir to coat shrimp and beans with vinaigrette. Pour warm vinaigrette over spinach and toss quickly. Plate the spinach and arrange shrimp and green beans on top.

Serves 4. 310 Calories per serving.

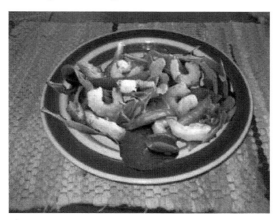

Diet Tip of the Day: After company leaves, have them take some of the leftover food (particularly the dessert) with them – or take the leftovers to work the next day.

Day 23 - Recipe
Beans & Greens Salad

⅓ cup chopped oregano
⅓ cup chopped parsley
3 cloves garlic, chopped
1 lemon, juiced
Prepare dressing by combining above ingredients and stirring in ¼ cup extra-virgin olive oil. Salt and black pepper to taste.
½ pound mesclun mix
¼ pound green beans
19-oz can garbanzo beans (chickpeas)
Arrange mesclun mix, garbanzo beans and green beans on large platter. Drizzle dressing over beans and greens.
Serves 4. Approximately 260 Calories per serving.

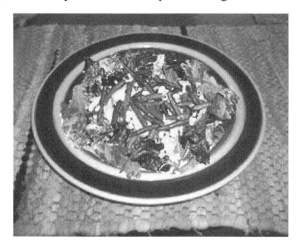

Diet Tip of the Day: Beans are a wonderful food but **beans are an incomplete protein**. If however beans are eaten with a whole-grain bread, the combination forms a complete protein – just as complete and nutritious as meat, poultry, or fish.

Day 24- Recipe

<u>Four-Bean Plus Salad</u> (This is a side dish)

Note that the total caloric value of the salad will change very little, if the proportions of the bean varieties and corn are varied – according to taste.

½ cup canned red kidney beans, drained and rinsed
½ cup canned black beans, drained and rinsed
½ cup canned chick peas, drained and rinsed
½ cup canned cannelloni beans, drained and rinsed
½ cup canned corn, drained
1 small red pepper, chopped
1 small green pepper, chopped
2 tablespoons extra-virgin olive oil
2 tablespoons lemon juice

In a large bowl mix red kidney beans, black beans, chick peas, cannelloni beans, corn and chopped red and green peppers. Stir in olive oil and lemon juice and plate.

<u>Serves about 6</u>. One serving is ½ cup – with about 135 Calories per serving

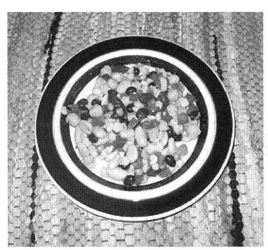

<u>Diet Tip of the Day:</u> Vigorous exercise doesn't necessarily stimulate you to overeat. Just the opposite. In many cases, exercise actually helps curb your appetite – immediately following a workout.

Day 25 - Recipe

Pan-Broiled Hanger Steak

1¼ pounds hanger steak, well trimmed of fat
¼ cup lime juice
8 small new potatoes, peeled and halved
½ pint cherry tomatoes (about 15), halved
Season both sides of steak with salt and pepper and place in sealable plastic bag with lime juice. Refrigerate for about one hour.

Boil potatoes about 10 minutes. Rinse in cold water. Sauté potatoes in small amount of vegetable oil over medium-high heat until brown.

Sauté cherry tomatoes in small amount of olive oil over medium-high heat until skin begins to crack. Season with chopped fresh basil.

Heat a skillet over medium-high heat. Sear hanger steak on one side for about 5 minutes. Turn over and sear other side approximately 5 minutes (for medium done). Pour off any fat that may have accumulated. Cut into ½-inch slices.
Serves 4. About 320 Calories per serving (for the hanger steak only)

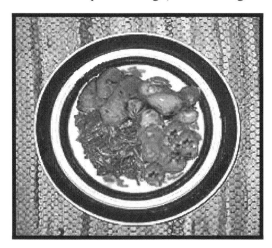

Diet Tip of the Day: If you go to a **party**, don't stand near the food! Be aware of the temptation. Make the effort, and you'll find you eat less.

Day 26 - Recipe
Tina's Grilled Scallops &Polenta

1 pound sea scallops
¾ cup polenta cornmeal
¾ cup skim milk
1 medium portobello mushroom
½ pound green beans
¼ cup chopped red onion
16 asparagus spear
1 teaspoon extra-virgin olive oil

Bring 1½ cups of water and skim milk to rapid boil. Add salt to taste and slowly add polenta while stirring. Reduce heat. Continue stirring until desired consistency is reached. Pour polenta into lightly greased pan. After polenta has cooled cover and refrigerate. Cut chilled polenta into 4 pieces. Grill on medium-hot fire – about two minutes on each side.

Brush portobello mushroom and asparagus spear with olive oil and place on grill for about 3 minutes on each side.

Grill scallops on medium-hot fire. Turn after two minutes or when first side turns opaque. Grill until second side turns opaque – about another 2 minutes. Don't overcook but test a scallop by cutting to make sure it's cooked through. Salt and pepper to taste.

Serves 4. The food on the plate pictured below totals about 380 Calories.

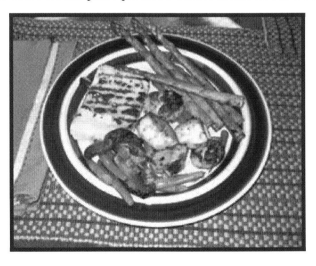

Diet Tip of the Day: To have better control of what you eat **bring your lunch to work**.

Day 27 - Recipe

Fettuccine in Summer Sauce

This sauce is often served in the summer because it's lighter than what is usually dished up with pasta. But despite its name the sauce is wonderful year round.

½ lb fettuccine
8 oz fresh asparagus, trimmed & cut in 2-inch pieces
¾ pint cherry tomatoes (about 20), halved
2 Tbsp plus 1 tsp extra-virgin olive oil, divided
2 cloves of garlic, chopped
½ small onion, diced

Cook fettuccine according to package directions. Drain and return pasta to pot; add a teaspoon of the olive oil and toss to coat. Meanwhile steam asparagus and drain.

In large skillet over medium-high heat, sauté cherry tomatoes in remaining 2 tablespoons of olive oil until skin begins to crack. Add onion and cook until translucent. Stir in garlic. Thin sauce with pasta liquid to desired consistency. Toss cooked pasta and asparagus into sauce and serve immediately.

Serves 4. About 290 Calories per serving

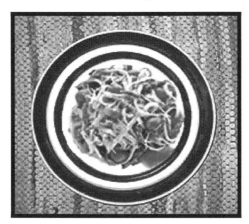

Diet Tip of the Day: A major weight-loss fallacy is that you can **get rid of abdominal fat** by working your abdominal muscles. This is based on the incorrect belief that fat is eliminated from a particular part of your body if you engage the muscles underneath that layer of fat. No such luck.

Day 28 - Recipe
Frozen Chicken Dinner

No recipe today. No cooking today. Another day off! There are plenty of frozen chicken choices in your local supermarket. Here are some reasonably good selections:

Poultry	Crustless Chicken Pot Pie	Smart Ones	~~200~~ 190
Poultry	Buffalo Style Chicken	Lean Cuisine	~~200~~ 190
Poultry	Home Style Chicken & Potatoes	Healthy Choice	200
Poultry	Honey Balsamic Chicken	Healthy Choice	210
Poultry	Sesame Stir Fry with Chicken	Lean Cuisine	280
Poultry	Roasted Turkey Breast	Lean Cuisine	~~280~~ 290
Poultry	Apple Cranberry Chicken	Lean Cuisine	280
Poultry	Chicken Fettuccini Alfredo	Healthy Choice	280
Poultry	Grilled Chicken Marinara	Healthy Choice	280
Poultry	Sweet & Spicy Orange Chicken	Healthy Choice	280
Poultry	Chicken Parmesan	Smart Ones	280
Poultry	Turkey Breast with Stuffing	Smart Ones	280

If you fall short of the **300 Calories allocated for today's frozen meal**. In this case, use the remaining calories anyway you wish. Overindulge on extra dessert or save the calories for another day.

See **Appendix A** on page 197 for our comprehensive list of frozen entrees. Please read the important **Frozen-Food Safety Warning** in **Appendix C** on page 203.

<u>**Diet Tip of the Day:**</u> The **general weight-change rule is "last on first off."** Assume as you gained weight, the first place you noticed it was on your thighs, next your buttocks, then your face. As you lose weight, it generally will come off in the reverse order, first from your face, then your rear and finally your thighs. And there is not much you can do about that. The truth is there is no food, no exercise, no magic belt, and no pill that will cause your body to lose fat in one place rather than another.

Day 29 - Recipe
Barbequed Shrimp & Corn

1½ pounds large shrimp, peeled and de-veined
3 Tbsp of your favorite bottled barbeque sauce
4 medium ears of corn

Pour barbeque sauce into shallow bowl. Toss shrimp in barbeque sauce to coat. Place shrimp on medium-hot grill. Turn shrimp after about two minutes or when shrimp turn pink. Grill until second side turns pink – approximately another 2 minutes. Don't overcook but test a shrimp by cutting to make sure it is cooked through. Salt and pepper to taste. Serve hot or at room temperature.

Serves 4. About 160 Calories per serving (shrimp only).

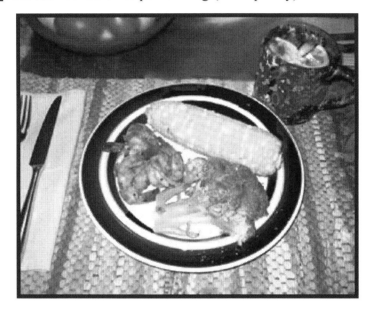

Diet Tip of the Day: A very **important weight-profile parameter** is your waist-to-hip ratio. Health risks for heart attack and stroke increase considerably for men with a ratio above 1.0 and for women with a ratio above 0.8. To calculate your ratio, measure your waist size (at its narrowest circumference) and divide it by your hip size (at the widest section).

Day 30 - Recipe

Cheeseburger Heaven

There's really not much to grilling hamburgers. The ideal meat for a juicy burger is ground chuck with about 20% fat, but we are talking diet here. So we opt for leaner, much leaner meat.

1¼ pounds ground sirloin (95% lean)
4 thin slices low-fat American cheese

Mix ground beef in large bowl. Salt and pepper to taste. Divide into 4 equal portions and form burgers about 1-inch thick.

Cook burgers over a hot fire on charcoal or gas-fired grill. For medium, cook about 4 minutes on each side. Top with slice of cheese. Add lettuce and tomato. Season to taste.

Serves 4. About 370 Calories per serving (cheeseburger only).

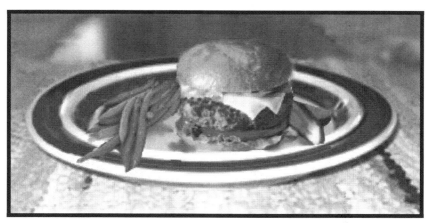

Diet Tip of the Day: **Plan to be on a diet the rest of your life**. Not necessarily a weight-reducing diet. At some point you'll want to just maintain your weight. But you will still need to continue to make good healthy food choices – and not slip back to your old eating habits.

Day 31 - Recipe

Tina's Baked Sea Bass

4 4-ounce Chilean sea bass fillets
½ pound green beans
¾ pint cherry tomatoes (about 20)
¾ cup brown rice (prepare per package directions)
Sea Bass: Dust filets with flour. Dip in egg wash & then Panko bread crumbs. Place fillets in baking dish coated with non-stick spray. Bake about 15 minutes in oven preheated to 350 °F.
Green Beans & Tomato: Place green beans in skillet. Add ¼-inch of water and cook over medium heat until water boils off. Add cherry tomatoes and olive oil. Stir well and sauté for a few minutes. Season with fresh rosemary and oregano.
Brown Rice-Pesto mix: Prepare brown rice per package directions. Add 4 teaspoons packaged "green" pesto. Mix thoroughly.
Red Pepper Sauce: Blend one roasted red pepper (skinned), ½ cup non-fat yogurt, 1 tsp lemon juice, 1 Tbsp olive oil, 1 Tbsp chili sauce, and a dash of Worcestershire sauce.
Serves 4. One plate consisting of one sea bass fillet with spooned over red pepper sauce (150 Calories), green beans & tomato mix (75 Calories), brown rice-pesto mix (120 Calories) and half ear of corn (50 Calories) – totals about 395 Calories.

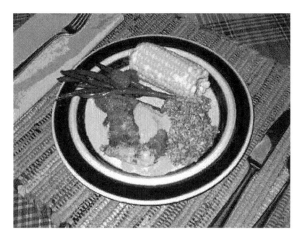

Diet Tip of the Day: Protein foods make you **feel full longer** and help prevent overeating.

Day 32 - Recipe
Turkey Tenders & Vegetables

2   turkey breast tenderloins (about 1½ lb)
1   medium eggplant (about ¾ lb)
¾   pound yellow (summer) squash
2   medium plum tomatoes, quartered

Marinade: Whisk in a bowl 2 tsp lemon zest, ¼ cup lemon juice, 2 Tbsp olive oil, 1 Tbsp chopped garlic, 1 Tbsp chopped rosemary, ¼ tsp salt and a pinch of black pepper. Put marinade and turkey breasts in large re-sealable plastic bag. Refrigerate about 45 minutes

Slice eggplant and squash lengthwise about ½-inch thick. Place with tomatoes on a baking sheet coated with a nonstick spray.

Grill turkey breasts approximately 7 to 9 minutes per side, or until an instant-read thermometer inserted from the side to middle registers 160°F. Slice turkey and set aside.

Grill eggplant and zucchini about 4 minutes per side, or until just tender. Grill tomatoes about 2 minutes per side, or until charred but not soft. Cut vegetables bite-size and toss with remaining marinade. Serve with sliced turkey.

Serves 4. About 350 Calories per serving (includes turkey and veggies)

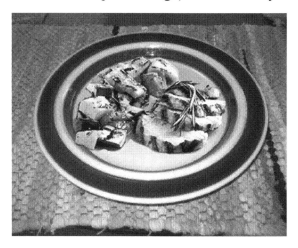

Diet Tip of the Day: It's a lot easier to eat 1000 Calories than it is to burn 1000 Calories exercising. So a stroll after dinner isn't going to offset the calories you ingested eating a Big Mac plus fries.

Day 33 - Recipe

Frozen-Fish Dinner

No recipe today. No cooking today. It's your day off! Some reasonably good frozen fish dinners are:

Seafood	Shrimp Alfredo	Lean Cuisine	~~230~~ 240
Seafood	Tuna Noodle Casserole	Smart Ones	~~250~~ 270
Seafood	Shrimp & Angel Hair Pasta	Lean Cuisine	~~280~~ 290
Seafood	Parmesan Crusted Fish	Lean Cuisine	~~290~~ 300
Seafood	Tortilla Crusted Fish	Lean Cuisine	~~300~~ 310

That's it. At this writing, there are just not that many frozen fish dinners for sale at supermarkets, although new entrees are being introduced continually. If you choose any of the above entrees, you will not use all of the **340 Calories allocated for this meal**. In this case, use the excess calories anyway you wish. Splurge on extra dessert or save the calories for another day!

See **Appendix A** on page 197 for our comprehensive list of frozen entrees. Please read the important **Frozen-Food Safety Warning** in **Appendix C** on page 203.

Diet Tip of the Day: It's amazing how many people tend to confuse thirst with hunger. This often results in overeating when actually drinking water might be the solution. So, the next time you have a seemingly uncontrollable food craving, try drinking a glass of water instead.

Day 34 - Recipe

Pasta Rapini

2 cloves garlic - coarsely chopped
1½ cups of crushed San Marzano tomatoes
2 cups Rapini (broccoli rabe)
1 tablespoon crushed red pepper flakes (optional)
½ pound medium-sized whole wheat pasta

Tomato Sauce: In large pan, sauté two tablespoons olive oil over medium-high heat. Add the garlic and sauté until translucent (but not browned). Add crushed San Marzano tomatoes (use plum tomatoes if San Marzano are not available) and bring to a boil. Reduce heat to low and simmer for about 30 minutes or until cooked. Season with salt and pepper. Set aside.

Rapini: Discard the tough stems and slice into 2-inch pieces. Bring a pot of water to a boil. Add Rapini (a variety of the vegetable broccoli rabe) and 1 tablespoon salt. Blanch Rapini about 5 minutes or until slightly cooked but still crunchy at stems. Drain, set aside and cover.

Cook pasta according to package instructions until al dente. Three minutes before pasta is ready, add the Rapini to the sauté pan (containing the tomato sauce). Heat mixture over medium heat. Drain pasta and add it to the pan with the Rapini and tomatoes. Add hot pepper flakes (optional) and toss for 1 to 2 minutes over high heat. Drizzle lightly with extra virgin olive oil and plate. Delicious!

Serves 4. About 290 Calories per serving

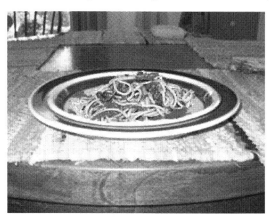

Diet Tip of the Day: Keep a daily food log to **record everything you eat**. For some people it really works wonders.

Day 35 - Recipe

Chicken Dinner - Out

No recipe today. No cooking today. Have a chicken dinner at your favorite restaurant, but make sure you choose a restaurant where you have a fighting chance to achieve your calorie goal. For your chicken dinner out, your maximum allowable calories (includes appetizer, soup, main course and dessert) are as follows:

- For the **1200 Calorie Diet**: 530 Calories
- For the **1500 Calorie Diet**: 630 Calories
- For the **1800 Calorie Diet**: 630 Calories

Tips for Eating Chicken Out: First, order simple and order skinless white meat only, such as broiled chicken breast with steamed vegetables and brown rice. (Incidentally, feel free to substitute skinless white meat turkey for chicken.) Tell the waiter you want no sauce, no gravy, nothing added. Then, knowing your calorie objective, and that chicken is about 50 Calories per ounce, most steamed vegetable servings average approximately 50 Calories per cup, and rice is about 100 Calories per ½ cup, decide how much to eat – and take the remainder home. If fresh fruit is not an option, pass on dessert and have the evening snack specified for that day in this diet.

In a restaurant, some nutritionists recommend you eat the low-calorie items on your plate first. Start with the salad, soup and veggies. By the time you get to the chicken and starches you will hopefully be full enough to be content with smaller portions of the higher-calorie choices.

Finally, some dieticians advise their dieting clients not to eat out. That's right. They believe eating at home is safer. But our thought is you have to eat out eventually so why not learn how while your resolve is high?

Diet Tip of the Day: To determine your frame size, circle your wrist with your thumb and third finger. If the tips of your fingers overlap, you have a small frame. If they just touch you are medium, and if they don't touch you have a large frame.

Day 36 - Recipe

Grilled Tilapia

Tilapia is a mild, white fish that inhabits fresh water. This fish has very low levels of mercury because it's fast-growing, short-lived, and mostly eats a vegetarian diet. According to the Monterey Bay Aquarium, choose tilapia farmed in the U.S., in environmentally friendly systems. "Avoid" farmed tilapia from China and Taiwan, where pollution and weak management are a problem.

4 Tilapia filets (about 6 ounces each)

Marinade: ¾ cup olive oil, ½ lemon, juiced, 1 tablespoons oregano, ½ teaspoon black pepper, ¼ cup red wine vinegar, ½ cup finely chopped parsley, 2 cloves garlic, minced and 2 dashes Tabasco (optional).

Combine all ingredients (except filets) in a large re-sealable plastic bag and shake well. Then place fish filets in the marinade for 30 minutes. Remove fillets from marinade and cook on hot grill for approximately 2 to 3 minutes per side.

Serves 4. About 300 Calories per serving (fish only)

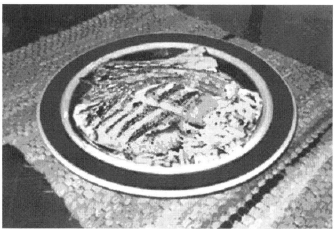

Photo shows two fish filets. Actual serving size is <u>one filet</u>.

Diet Tip of the Day: One serving of asparagus can provide you with 66% of your daily folate needs. Folate is a B-vitamin which is involved with cellular division, and therefore aids the development of a baby's nervous system.

Day 37 - Recipe
Lo-Cal Beef Stew

½ lb beef stew meat, fat trimmed & cut in 1" cubes
2 celery stalks diced
1 medium onion diced
3 large carrots cut into large chunks
3 large boiling potatoes, peeled & cut in chunks
½ up green beans
1 container beef stock (low sodium)
2 tablespoons of flour, and 1 tablespoon of olive oil
½ teaspoon dried herbs, and 1 bay leaf

Season meat with ½ teaspoon dried herbs, salt and pepper. In a Dutch oven, add olive oil and heat until warm. Add meat, diced onion and celery and cook over medium heat about 5 minutes. Add enough beef stock to cover meat. Bring to a boil. Reduce heat, add bay leaf, cover and simmer over low heat until meat is fork tender (about 1½ hours). Add potatoes and carrots. Cover and cook until vegetables are tender (about 30 min). Add green beans and cook an additional 10 min. Skim off any fat from the surface.

In a small bowl, add small amount of water to 2 tablespoons of flour – and stir. Pour the flour-water mixture into the stew and stir until a thick gravy forms. Taste and adjust seasoning. Spoon approximately ¼ of the stew in each plate.

Serves 4. About 365 Calories per serving

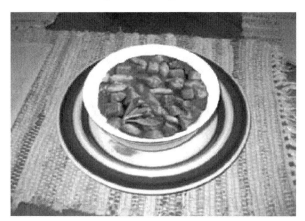

Diet Tip of the Day: Free-range animals get more exercise and eat a natural diet, so their meat is usually lower in fat and calories than farm-raised cattle.

Day 38 - Recipe

Pan-Broiled Lamb Chop

Pan broiling is a quick, easy and a relatively low-calorie technique that can be used to cook many meats.

Start with a rib lamb chop about ¾-inch thick that weighs roughly 6 ounces. Next, it is very important to carefully trim all the visible fat. (After removing the fat and accounting for the bone, about 4 ounces of lean meat should remain.)

Season the chop with salt and ground black pepper. Heat a well-seasoned cast iron or nonstick skillet over high heat. Add the chop (or chops) and cook approximately 4 minutes on each side. (Check center of chop with a small incision to determine when the meat is done.) Plate and serve immediately.

Serves 1: About 320 Calories per chop

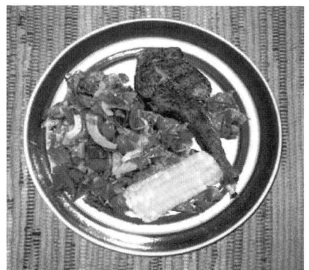

Note corn-on-the-cob is only for the 1800-Calorie diet.

Diet Tip of the Day: According to a study published in the Journal of Food Chemistry, broccoli, spinach, kale, Brussels sprouts and other dark green vegetables have the highest cancer-fighting potential found in produce.

Day 39 - Recipe

Chicken with Veggies

  4 boneless, skinless chicken breast halves (about 5 oz each)
  12 broccoli florets
  1 bunch of asparagus
  2 ripe medium-size tomatoes
  2 tablespoons Lo-Cal (light) salad dressing

Place evenly cut broccoli and asparagus spear in a microwave-safe pan, add a little water to bottom of the pan and top with microwave-safe plastic wrap. (Be sure to pull back one corner of the plastic topper so some steam can escape.) Check veggies periodically and take them out of the microwave when they reach desired softness.

Season chicken breasts evenly with salt and pepper. Heat a large nonstick skillet over medium-high heat. Coat pan with cooking spray. Cook chicken about 4 minutes on each side or until no pink remains.

For each serving, plate one chicken breast and a portion of the steamed broccoli and asparagus. Add one-half of a tomato cut into pieces. Drizzle about 2 tablespoons of a light salad dressing that contains no more than 50 Calories in 2 tablespoons.

Serves 4: One serving of chicken breast halve, veggies & dressing is about 365 Calories.

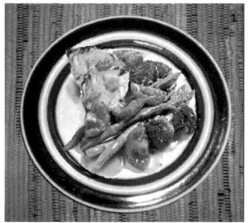

Shown drizzled with Light Thousand Island dressing.

Diet Tip of the Day: Steaming in a microwave oven is one of the best ways to cook veggies so they retain nutrients. Another advantage is the cooking adds no fat or sodium.

Day 40 - Recipe
Fish Dinner - Out

No recipe today. No cooking today. Have a fish dinner at your favorite restaurant, but make sure you choose a restaurant where you have a good chance to achieve your calorie goal. For today, your **goal for dinner is a maximum of 595 Calories**. This includes appetizer, soup, main course and dessert.

Tips for Eating Fish Out: The following is almost an exact repeat of the advice given eating out on previous days. First, order simple, such as broiled fish with steamed vegetables and brown rice. Tell the waiter you want no sauce, no gravy, nothing added. Then, knowing your calorie objective, and that fish is about 50 Calories per ounce, most steamed vegetable servings average approximately 50 Calories per cup, and rice is about 100 Calories per ½ cup, decide how much to eat – and take the remainder home. If fresh fruit is not an option, pass on dessert and have the evening snack specified for that day in the diet.

In a restaurant, some nutritionists recommend you eat the low-calorie items on your plate first. Start with the salad, soup and veggies. By the time you get to the fish and starches you will hopefully be full enough to be content with smaller portions of the higher-calorie choices.

Diet Tip of the Day: The average egg has only 210 mg of cholesterol (found in the yoke), contains 80 calories, many vitamins many minerals. If you're healthy and your LDL blood cholesterol level is low, many experts feel you can safely eat one egg per day.

Day 41 - Recipe
Pasta e Fagioli

This is one variation of a traditional, nutritious peasant dish served all over Italy.

14.5-oz can whole tomatoes with juice, crushed
14.5-oz can cannellini beans, drained
1 cup of any tube-shaped pasta
2 tablespoon olive oil
1 medium onion, diced
2 cloves garlic, minced
1 stalk celery, finely chopped
3 cups chicken stock
2 cups fresh baby spinach or escarole
1 tsp dried basil
½ teaspoon dried oregano
2 Tbsp fresh parsley, chopped

Heat olive oil, onion and celery in large saucepan over medium heat. Sauté until onions are golden brown. Add garlic and stir constantly for one minute. Pour in tomatoes and their juices and bring to a boil. Add beans and chicken stock and return to a boil. Stir in spinach (or escarole) and seasonings. Simmer for about 5 minutes. Add pasta and cook about 15 minutes or until pasta is tender but firm. If needed, thin soup with hot water.

Ladle into soup bowls. Garnish with grated Parmesan cheese. Salt and pepper to taste.
Serves 4. About 300 Calories per serving.

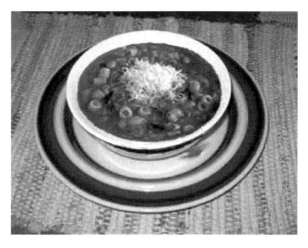

Day 42 - Recipe
Dawn's Blueberry Muffins

Wholesome whole-wheat blueberry muffins just like grandma used to make. Serve them at breakfast, or as a nutritious dessert, or a wonderful snack. (Make a dozen. Have one today and store the remainder in your freezer until they are called for again later in the diet.)

4 ounces bran flakes
¼ cup sugar
1¼ cups whole wheat flour
1 teaspoon baking soda
¼ teaspoon baking powder
¼ teaspoon salt
½ cup blueberries (fresh or frozen)
1 egg, beaten
1 cup buttermilk
¼ cup vegetable oil

Preheat oven to 400 °F. Coat muffin tins with nonstick cooking spray. In a bowl combine dry ingredients. In another bowl combine wet ingredients and mix thoroughly. Add wet ingredients to dry ingredients and mix until just blended. Do not over mix. Gently fold in blueberries. Spoon batter into muffin tins until two-thirds full. Bake 15 minutes or until muffin tops are golden brown.

Yield is 12 Muffins, 145 Calories each

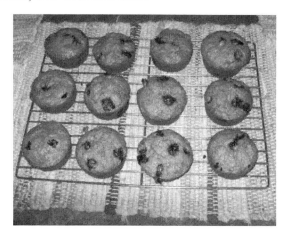

Diet Tip of the Day: **Acquire a good low-calorie cookbook**. Be sure the recipes cover breakfast, lunch and dinner, and all the recipes contain nutritional information, especially the calories per serving.

Day 43 - Recipe

Beef Kebob

1 lb boneless beef tenderloin steaks, 1" thick
8 ounces medium mushrooms
2 medium bell peppers (any color), cut in pieces
Marinate ingredients:
2 tablespoons olive oil
1 tablespoon chopped fresh oregano
2 cloves garlic, minced
½ teaspoon ground black pepper

Cut beef steak into 1-inch square pieces. Combine marinate ingredients in large bowl. Add beef, mushrooms and bell pepper pieces. Toss to coat. Cover bowl and refrigerate for about two hours. Thread beef and vegetable pieces onto eight 12-inch metal skewers.

Grill kebobs over medium-high heat for 8 to 10 minutes, turning occasionally. Check center of meat with a small incision to determine when the meat is done.

Microwave a one-pound package of frozen mixed vegetables. Plate two kebob skewers and about one-quarter of the mixed veggies.
Serves 4. One plate consisting of two kebob skewers (350 Calories) plus ¼ pound of mixed green vegetables (40 Calories) totals about 390 Calories.

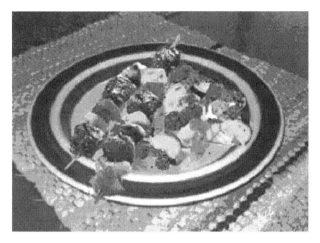

Diet Tip of the Day: Remember your stomach is about the size of your fist. So it doesn't take much food to fill it comfortably.

Day 44 - Recipe

Baked Haddock

4   4-oz haddock fillets (or salmon fillets)
½   cup white wine
½   cup non-fat yogurt mixed with ¼ cup pureed roasted red pepper
½   pound green beans
¾   pint cherry tomatoes (about 20)
1   tablespoon olive oil
¾   cup bulgur, prepared per package directions

Lightly dust fillets with flour. Dip in beaten egg white and then in Panko bread crumbs. Brown fillets in non-stick pan. Place fillets skin side down in baking dish coated with non-stick spray. Add white wine and cook in oven preheated to 350 °F for about 15 minutes. Spoon pan juices over fillets. Salt and pepper to taste.

Place green beans in skillet. Add ¼-inch of water and cook over medium heat until water boils off. Add cherry tomatoes and olive oil. Stir well and sauté for a few minutes. Season with fresh rosemary and oregano. Salt and pepper to taste.

Plate haddock fillet and spoon over yogurt-red pepper sauce. Garnish with fresh parsley. Add green beans & tomato mix and the bulgur. Serve hot.

Serves 4. One plate consisting of one haddock fillet (215 Calories) with green beans & tomato mix (65 Calories) and bulgur (140 Calories) totals 420 Calories.

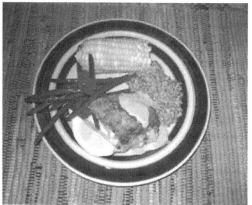

Note that corn-on-the-cob is only for the 1800 Calorie diet.

Diet Tip of the Day: It's much easier to stay with an exercise program when it's done in tandem. So enlist a friend to be your exercise buddy.

Day 45 - Recipe
Chicken Cacciatore

¾ lb skinless, boneless chicken breast halves
¼ lb of your favorite pasta
½ cup chopped onion
½ cup chopped green bell pepper
14.5-ounce can chopped tomatoes, drained
8-ounce can tomato sauce
1½ teaspoons Italian seasoning
⅓ cup sliced ripe olives
⅛ teaspoon black pepper

Cut chicken breasts into small pieces. Spray a large heavy skillet with olive oil flavored cooking spray.

Sauté chicken, onion and green pepper for 6 to 8 minutes. Stir in drained tomatoes and tomato sauce. Add Italian seasoning, olives and ⅛ teaspoon ground black pepper. Mix well to combine. Lower heat and simmer for 15 to 20 minutes, stirring occasionally.

Cook pasta per package directions. Ladle chicken and sauce over pasta and serve immediately.
Serves 4. About 310 Calories per serving

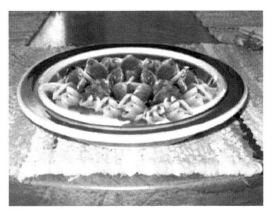

Diet Tip of the Day: Inevitably, you're going to be faced with a stressful situation. Instead of turning to food for comfort, be prepared with some non-food tactics that work for you, such as listening to music, reading, writing in a journal, or meditating.

Day 46 - Recipe
Poached Cod in Tomato Broth

2   cups dry white wine
1   cup clam juice
2   cans (14.5-ounce) diced tomatoes, drained
1   small onion, diced
1   garlic clove, minced
½   tsp dried parsley, or sprigs of fresh parsley
1   bay leaf
12 black olives, pitted and halved
4   cod fish fillets (about 6 ounces each)
Note that sole, flounder, halibut or haddock may be substituted for cod.

Use a pan large enough to hold the fish in a single layer. Place all the ingredients except the fish in the pan. Over high heat, bring poaching liquid to a boil (pan uncovered). Reduce heat and simmer the liquid another 6 minutes.

Carefully place the fish filets in the liquid. Cover the pan and reduce heat until liquid is just simmering. Poach until fish are completely opaque and tender – about 8 minutes. Plate fish and ladle broth over fish.
Serves 4. 275 Calories per serving.

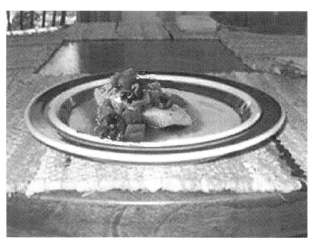

Diet Tip of the Day: A **good reducing diet must help you remain healthy** while you are losing weight.

Day 47 - Recipe

<u>Chinese Dinner - Out</u>

No recipe today. No cooking today. Have a Chinese dinner at your favorite restaurant, but make sure you choose a restaurant where you have a reasonable chance to achieve your calorie goal. For today, **your goal for dinner is a maximum of 640 Calories**. This includes any appetizer, soup, main course and any dessert.

Tips for Eating Chinese: You can consume a lot of calories in a Chinese restaurant – if you order carelessly. For example a typical portion of General Tso's chicken is loaded with about 1,000 Calories, then add another 200 Calories for a cup of rice.

First rule, order simple. Look for an entree with lots of vegetables, some fish or chicken and brown rice. Tell the waiter you want your food steamed with any sauce on the side. (This is not only a low-calorie way of eating Chinese food but is also the most nutritious way to eat Chinese food.)

Then, knowing your 640 Calorie objective, and that chicken and fish are about 50 Calories per ounce, most steamed vegetable servings average approximately 50 Calories per cup, and rice is about 200 Calories per cup, decide how much of the meal you can eat – and take the remainder home. (Note that you will be eating half a serving of left over Chinese food for lunch tomorrow.) To stay within your maximum allowable calorie total, you should pass on dessert and have the evening snack specified for that day in the diet.

Incidentally, although Chinese is specified, feel free to substitute Thai food, Vietnamese, Indian, Middle Eastern, or any other favorite ethnic food. Just make sure you don't exceed the maximum allowable 640 calories for this meal.

<u>Diet Tip of the Day:</u> Inevitably, everyone on a diet hits a frustrating **weight-loss plateau**. Two ways to bust through the plateau are: first to reduce your calorie intake and second to step up your exercise intensity.

Day 48 - Recipe

Healthy Pasta Salad

½ pound fusilli pasta, cooked until tender but firm
2 broccoli crowns, chopped
¼ pint cherry tomatoes (about 8), halved
½ cup black olives, halved
½ cup garbanzo beans (chick peas)
½ cup fresh "light" mozzarella, chopped
1 tablespoon basil
1 tablespoon rosemary
2 teaspoons garlic powder
¼ cup of a **recommended dressing** (see page 10)

Combine dry ingredients in a medium-size bowl. Stir in salad dressing. Mix thoroughly. Salt and black pepper to taste.

Serves 4. 370 Calories per serving.

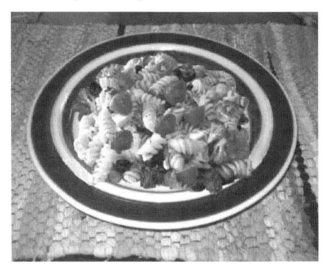

Diet Tip of the Day: Ask yourself: "**Why am I overweight**?" Do you eat too much of everything? Too much dessert? Drink too much beer? Is your only exercise walking from the TV to the refrigerator? Determine the why and then focus on one or two of your problem areas. Sometimes it's that simple.

Day 49 - Recipe
Frozen-Meat Dinner

No recipe today. No cooking today. Another day off! That's it. At this writing, there are just not that many frozen meat dinners for sale at supermarkets, although new entrees are being introduced continually. Here are some reasonably good frozen-meat dinners:

Meat	Steak Portobella	Lean Cuisine	160
Meat	Asian Style Beef & Broccoli	Smart Ones	~~160~~ 170
Meat	Beef Merlot	Healthy Choice	180
Meat	Home style Beef Pot Roast	Smart Ones	180
Meat	Salisbury Steak with Mac & Cheese	Lean Cuisine	~~270~~ 290
Pasta	Pasta with Swedish Meatballs	Smart Ones	~~280~~ 290
Meat	Classic Meat Loaf	Healthy Choice	300

If you choose any of the above entrees, you will fall short of the **300 Calories allocated for this day**. In this case, use the remaining calories anyway you wish. Indulge on extra dessert or save the calories for another day.

See **Appendix A** on page 197 for our comprehensive list of frozen entrees. Please read the important **Frozen-Food Safety Warning** in **Appendix C** on page 203.

Diet Tip of the Day: Experts agree that whether you are trying to lose weight or just maintain your weight, **it's calories that count**. It doesn't matter what foods the calories are from. To lose weight you must eat fewer calories than you burn. Calories count! Not carbs, not Weight Watchers points. Calories – period!

Pan-Fried Sole

4   sole fillets (6-ounces each), skinned
1   tablespoon olive oil
Salsa Ingredients:
1 pint cherry tomatoes, quartered
¾ cup cucumber, finely chopped
⅓ cup yellow bell pepper, finely chopped
3 tablespoons fresh basil, chopped
2 tablespoons capers
1½ tablespoons shallots, finely chopped
1 tablespoon balsamic vinegar
2 teaspoons lemon rind, grated
Combine salsa ingredients in a bowl and stir in ½ teaspoon salt and ⅛ teaspoon black pepper. Mix thoroughly.

Heat olive oil in a large nonstick skillet over medium-high heat. Season sole fillets with ½ teaspoon salt and ⅛ teaspoon black pepper. Add fish to pan; cook about 1½ minutes on each side or until fish flakes easily when tested with a fork. Spoon salsa over fish and serve immediately.
Serves 4. 325 Calories per serving

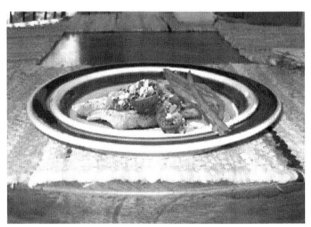

Diet Tip of the Day: If you are overweight start on a weight loss diet now because it will only become **more difficult to lose weight as you get older**.

Day 51 - Recipe

Beans & Greens Salad (Repeated)

⅓ cup chopped oregano
⅓ cup chopped parsley
3 cloves garlic, chopped
1 lemon, juiced
Prepare dressing by combining above ingredients and stirring in ¼ cup extra-virgin olive oil. Salt and pepper to taste.
½ pound mesclun mix
¼ pound green beans
19-ounce can garbanzo beans (chickpeas)
Arrange mesclun mix, garbanzo beans and green beans on a large platter. Drizzle dressing over beans and greens.
<u>Serves 4</u>. Approximately 260 Calories per serving.

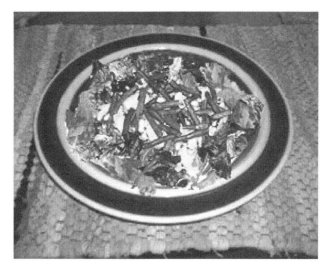

<u>Diet Tip of the Day:</u> **Fat-free isn't always your best bet**. Low fat doesn't necessarily mean low calorie! Most often sugar is substituted for fat and the calorie total remains the same or even higher. Instead, look for low-calorie or reduced-calorie foods.

Day 52 - Recipe

Chicken Piccata

1 pound boneless skinless chicken breast halves
2 teaspoons olive oil
1 teaspoon minced garlic
¼ cup shallots, diced
¾ pound fresh green beans, washed and snipped
1 teaspoon lemon juice
¼ cup capers, rinsed
2 fresh lemons, cut into small wedges

In a skillet, heat olive oil and minced garlic over medium heat. Sauté chicken breasts and shallots for two to three minutes, tossing often, until chicken is partially cooked. Add green beans and one teaspoon of lemon juice and sauté for an additional two to three minutes, or until chicken is completely cooked and green beans are al dente. Add capers; and cover chicken. Let sit for one more minute to warm capers. Serve immediately with wedges of lemon.

Serves 4. 270 calories per serving

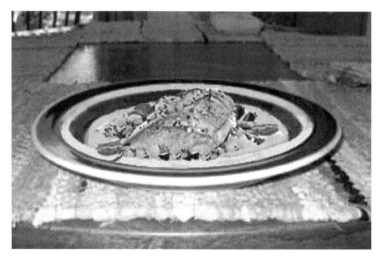

Diet Tip of the Day: Handle **occasional overeating by compensating**. To do this, estimate how far you have strayed from your weight-loss diet and then make amends at the next opportunity (usually the next meal or two) – by eating less.

Day 53 - Recipe

Beef Steak Strips

1 lb top loin sirloin, or top round about ¾" thick
1 tsp garlic, finely chopped
½ tsp dry thyme
½ tsp salt and ¼ tsp black peppercorns
Cut the steak into 3-inch long by ¼-inch thick strips Sprinkle the beef strips with garlic, thyme, salt and pepper. Prepare a large non-stick skillet over medium-high heat. Add the steak strips and shake the skillet constantly to avoid sticking. Cook approximately 2 to 3 minutes until meat is seared but pink inside. Check the center by making small incision.
Serves 4. About 330 Calories per serving (meat only).

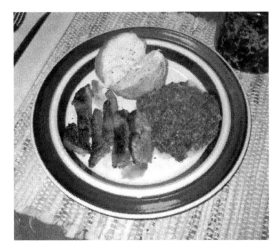

Diet Tip of the Day: Bear in mind, that knowledge and the discipline to **workout regularly** are far more important than fancy equipment.

Day 54 - Recipe
Tina's Grilled Scallops & Polenta

1 pound sea scallops
¾ cup polenta cornmeal
¾ cup skim milk
1 medium Portobello mushroom
½ pound green beans
¼ cup chopped red onion
16 asparagus spear
1 teaspoon extra-virgin olive oil

Bring 1½ cups of water and skim milk to rapid boil. Add salt to taste and slowly add polenta while stirring. Reduce heat. Continue stirring until desired consistency is reached. Pour polenta into lightly greased pan. After polenta has cooled cover and refrigerate. Cut chilled polenta into 4 pieces. Grill on medium-hot fire – about two minutes on each side.

Brush Portobello mushroom and asparagus spear with olive oil and place on grill for about 3 minutes on each side.

Grill scallops on medium-hot fire. Turn after two minutes or when first side turns opaque. Grill until second side turns opaque – about another 2 minutes. Don't overcook but test a scallop by cutting to make sure it's cooked through. Salt and pepper to taste.

<u>Serves 4</u>. The food on the plate pictured below totals about 380 Calories.

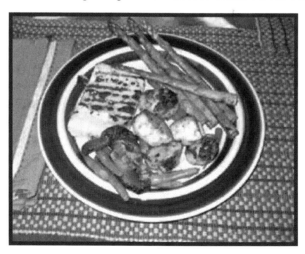

<u>Diet Tip of the Day:</u> To have better control of what you eat **bring your lunch to work**.

Day 55 - Recipe

Hearty Vegetable Soup

2 15-oz cans white kidney beans, drained
1 tablespoon olive oil
½ large yellow onion, chopped
2 garlic cloves, minced
1 cup chopped fresh tomatoes
2 celery stalks, cut into ½-inch pieces
1½ carrots, cut into ½-inch pieces
5 cups vegetable stock
1 medium potato, cut into ½-inch pieces
¼ cup chopped fresh basil
¼ head of red cabbage, cut into ½-inch pieces
2 zucchini or summer squash, cut into ½-inch pieces

Heat olive oil in a large pot over medium heat. Add onion and garlic.
Sauté 5 minutes. Add green cabbage, tomatoes, celery, and carrots. Sauté
10 minutes. Add beans, 5 cups of stock, potatoes, and basil. Bring to a
boil. Reduce heat, cover and simmer for one hour. Add red cabbage,
zucchini and salt . Cover and simmer until vegetables are tender, about 20
minutes longer. Stir in about ¼ cup Parmesan cheese and sprinkle a dash
of Tabasco hot sauce if you want a little zip

Serves 4. 360 Calories per serving

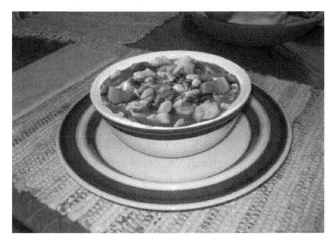

Diet Tip of the Day: Water and fiber contain no calories – that is **zero
Calories** per ounce.

Day 56 - Recipe
Frozen Chicken Dinner

No recipe today. No cooking today. Another day off! There are plenty of frozen chicken choices in your local supermarket. Here are some reasonably good selections:

Poultry	Crustless Chicken Pot Pie	Smart Ones	~~200~~ 190
Poultry	Buffalo Style Chicken	Lean Cuisine	~~200~~ 190
Poultry	Home Style Chicken & Potatoes	Healthy Choice	200
Poultry	Honey Balsamic Chicken	Healthy Choice	210
Poultry	Sesame Stir Fry with Chicken	Lean Cuisine	280
Poultry	Roasted Turkey Breast	Lean Cuisine	~~280~~ 290
Poultry	Apple Cranberry Chicken	Lean Cuisine	280
Poultry	Chicken Fettuccini Alfredo	Healthy Choice	280
Poultry	Grilled Chicken Marinara	Healthy Choice	280
Poultry	Sweet & Spicy Orange Chicken	Healthy Choice	280
Poultry	Chicken Parmesan	Smart Ones	280
Poultry	Turkey Breast with Stuffing	Smart Ones	280

If you choose the first four meals of the above, you will fall far short of the **300 Calories allocated for today's frozen meal**. In this case, use the remaining 100 or so calories anyway you wish. Splurge on extra dessert or save the calories for another day.

See **Appendix A** on page 197 for our comprehensive list of frozen entrees. Please read the important **Frozen-Food Safety Warning** in **Appendix C** on page 203.

Diet Tip of the Day: To prevent or delay the onset of type II diabetes, experts urge the overweight to lose weight and work out regularly. Weight loss helps your body use insulin more efficiently, and exercise helps metabolize excess circulating blood glucose.

Day 57 - Recipe

Salmon with Mango Salsa

4 salmon fillets (about 5 ounces each)
1½ pounds baby new potatoes, halved
1 mango, ripe
3 green onions, finely chopped
3 tablespoons chopped fresh cilantro
2 tablespoons lemon juice
2 teaspoons extra-virgin olive oil
4 cups watercress

Remove any tiny bones from salmon. Press crushed peppercorns into flesh side of salmon. Set aside. Place halved potatoes into saucepan. Cover with water and bring to a boil. Reduce the heat and simmer until tender, about 10-12 minutes and drain.

Prepare salsa: Peel and seed the mango. Dice the mango flesh and put into a large bowl. Mix in green onions, cilantro, lemon juice, olive oil, and an optional dash of Tabasco.

Heat a grill pan coated with nonstick cooking spray over medium-high heat. Place salmon fillets in pan, skin-side down. Cook for 4 minutes. Turn fish over and cook until done, about another 4 minutes. Arrange watercress and new potatoes on serving plates. Place salmon on top and spoon over mango salsa.

Serves 4. 460 Calories per serving

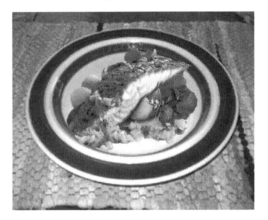

Diet Tip of the Day: All **foods are a combination of water, carbohydrate, protein, fat and fiber**. Knowing this can lead to a better understanding of why a food has a particular caloric value.

Day 58 - Recipe
Pork Chop with Orange Slices

4   loin pork chops, ½-inch-thick (about 1½ lbs total, including bones)
8   orange slices, ¼-inch-thick
1   teaspoon salt
¾   teaspoon black pepper
¼   cup orange marmalade preserve
½   cup bottled fruit-based barbecue sauce
such as Grandville's Gourmet BBQ Sauce
Marinade: ½ cup orange juice, 2 teaspoons soy sauce and ¼ teaspoon
crushed red pepper.

Combine pork chops and marinade in large re-sealable plastic bag.
Refrigerate for about 30 minutes. Remove chops from marinade and season
with salt and black pepper.

Stir together orange marmalade and BBQ sauce in a small bowl. Brush
one side of pork chops evenly with half of marmalade-BBQ mixture. Grill
chops, with marmalade-BBQ mixture side up over medium-high heat
(about 375°) for about 5 minutes or until done. Turn chops, and brush with
remaining marmalade-BBQ mixture. Grill another 5 minutes or until done.
Grill orange slices over medium-high heat, 1 minute on each side.
Serves 4. 470 Calories per serving (includes pork chop and orange slices).

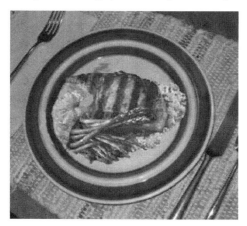

Diet Tip of the Day: Make sure fat is trimmed from meat. Most meats are
about 80 Calories per ounce – whereas, pure fat is 256 Calories per ounce!

Day 59 - Recipe

Fish Dinner - Out

No recipe today. No cooking today. Have a fish dinner at your favorite restaurant, but make sure you choose a restaurant where you have a good chance to achieve your calorie goal. For today, your **goal for dinner is a maximum of 595 Calories**. This includes appetizer, soup, main course and dessert.

Tips for Eating Fish Out: The following is almost an exact repeat of the advice given eating out on previous days. First order simple, such as broiled fish with steamed vegetables and brown rice. Tell the waiter you want no sauce, no gravy, nothing added. Then, knowing your calorie objective, and that fish is about 50 Calories per ounce, most steamed vegetable servings average approximately 50 Calories per cup, and rice is about 100 Calories per ½ cup, decide how much to eat – and take the remainder home. If fresh fruit is not an option, pass on dessert and have the evening snack specified for that day in the diet.

In a restaurant, some nutritionists recommend you eat the low-calorie items on your plate first. Start with the salad, soup and veggies. By the time you get to the fish and starches you will hopefully be full enough to be content with smaller portions of the higher-calorie choices.

Diet Tip of the Day: A handful of studies suggest that chewing gum may help reduce your craving for sweet snacks, and cut your caloric intake by about 50 per day. Another study actually showed that gum chewers experienced a small increase in their daily energy expenditure. And gum adds hardly any calories to your diet. Regular gum has about 10 calories and sugar-free varieties about five calories per stick.

Day 60 - Recipe

Chicken Stew over Rice

4   boneless skinless chicken breasts (about 1 lb)
1   medium Onion
3   stalks celery
12 mushrooms
2   cups baby carrots
3   cups broccoli florets
½   teaspoon black pepper
¼   teaspoon herb seasoning blend
2   teaspoons Worcestershire Sauce
1   bay leaf
1   cup Campbell's Cream of Chicken Soup

Prepare a large, heavy, stove-top pot with cooking spray. Sauté at medium-high heat finely chop onion until caramelized. Cut chicken into bite size pieces and add to pot. Cook and toss until chicken is no longer pink. Add black pepper, herb seasoning and Worcestershire sauce. Stir. Add sliced celery and mushrooms, and then broccoli, carrots and bay leaf. Pour in Cream of Chicken soup. Gradually add one cup water while stirring. (You may want to add more water to get consistency desired.) Simmer until hot and flavors have combined. Serve over rice.

Serves 4. 360 Calories per serving (not including the brown rice below the stew).

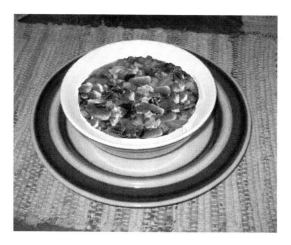

Diet Tip of the Day: Studies show people who eat 5 to 6 **mini-meals** and snacks a day don't feel as hungry and are better able to control their appetite and their weight.

Day 61 - Recipe

Shrimp over Spaghetti

½ lb spaghetti
1 lb shrimp, peeled and de-veined
6 ounces dry white wine
3 tablespoons olive oil
3 cloves garlic, sliced thin
¼ cup chopped basil leaves

Cook spaghetti according to package directions. Save ½ cup of the pasta cooking water.

In a large skillet over medium heat, cook olive oil and garlic, stirring until garlic turns golden, and then discard garlic. Add shrimp and increase heat to medium-high and stir in chopped basil leaves, white wine and ½ cup cooking water. Cook another 2 to 3 minutes or until shrimp are just firm. Spoon shrimp and sauce over spaghetti. Season with salt and black pepper. Garnish with parsley.

Serves 4. 450 Calories per serving

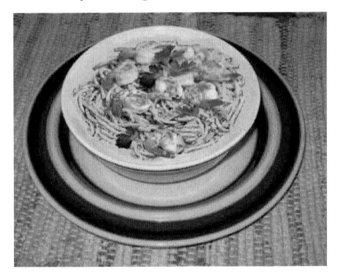

Diet Tip of the Day: If your caloric intake on a weight-loss diet is constant, your **rate of weight loss will decrease with time**. So if you want to lose weight at a constant rate over time, you must eat slightly less (or exercise harder) as you lose weight.

Beef Burgundy

1 lb boneless beef chuck, trimmed & cut in 1" pieces
2 large carrots, cut into 1-inch pieces
1 medium onion, cut into 1-inch pieces
1 tablespoon flour
1 tablespoon tomato paste
1 clove garlic, crushed
1 tablespoon olive oil
1 cup dry red wine
2 sprigs fresh thyme
10 ounces mushrooms, sliced in half
8 ounces frozen peas

In Dutch oven, heat oil on medium-high until hot. Add beef and cook 5 to 6 minutes or until beef is browned on all sides. Transfer beef to a bowl. Preheat oven to 325° F. To drippings in Dutch oven, add carrots, garlic, and onion. Stir occasionally and cook 10 minutes or until vegetables are browned and tender. Stir in flour, tomato paste, ½ teaspoon salt, and ¼ teaspoon black pepper, and cook another minute. Add wine and heat to boiling, stirring until browned bits are loosened from bottom of Dutch oven. Return meat and any juices in the bowl to Dutch oven. Add thyme and mushrooms; bring to a boil. Cover and bake 1½ hours or until meat is fork-tender. Discard thyme sprigs. Before stew is done, cook peas per package instructions and add peas to Dutch oven.

Serves 4. 350 Calories per serving

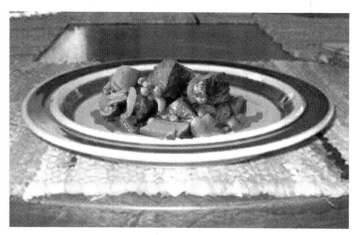

Day 63 - Recipe

Chicken Cutlet

Buy 4 skinless, boneless chicken cutlets or breast halves (about 1 lb), flattened to about ¼ to ½-inch thick.

¾ cup Panko bread crumbs
⅓ cup grated Parmesan cheese
1 egg, beaten
4 tablespoons extra-virgin olive oil, divided

Season chicken cutlets with salt and pepper. Combine bread crumbs and Parmesan cheese in a shallow bowl. Whisk egg in a separate shallow bowl. Dip chicken in egg and then coat both sides in crumb mixture.

Heat 2 tablespoons of olive oil in large skillet over medium-high heat. Add 2 cutlets, and cook 2 minutes on each side or until cooked through. Repeat with 2 tablespoons olive oil and remaining 2 cutlets. Serve hot. **Serves 4.** 450 Calories per serving (chicken cutlet only)

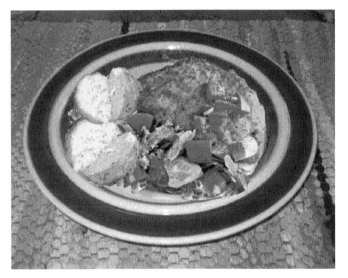

Diet Tip of the Day: **Working out at home** has some significant advantages. Your workout takes less time because you don't have to drive back and forth to a fitness facility; and you have the flexibility of dividing your workout into smaller time segments to fit your day, and working out at home is less expensive.

Day 64 - Recipe
Personal-Size Meat Loaf

1   pound extra lean ground beef
⅓   cup quick oats
2   egg whites
½   cup chipotle salsa, divided
¼   cup ketchup, divided

Place egg whites in a large bowl, mixing well with a whisk. Stir in oats, 6 tablespoons salsa, and 2 tablespoons ketchup. Add beef and mix well. Divide beef mixture into 4 equal portions, shaping each into an oval-shaped loaf. and place loaves on baking pan lined with tin foil and coated with cooking spray. Bake in preheated oven at 350°F for 30 minutes or until done.

Combine remaining 2 tablespoons salsa and 2 tablespoons ketchup in a small bowl. Spread mixture evenly over individual meat loaves.
Serves 4. 410 Calories per serving (meat loaf only)

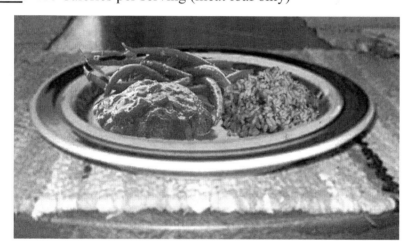

Diet Tip of the Day: To make sure you stay on track, **weigh in once a week**. There may be times when you might not see a weight loss, often because lost fat is temporarily replaced by water. This condition will gradually be corrected as you continue dieting.

Day 65 - Recipe

Frozen-Fish Dinner

No recipe today. No cooking today. It's your day off! Some reasonably good frozen fish dinners are:

Seafood	Shrimp Alfredo	Lean Cuisine	~~230~~ 240
Seafood	Tuna Noodle Casserole	Smart Ones	~~250~~ 270
Seafood	Shrimp & Angel Hair Pasta	Lean Cuisine	~~280~~ 290
Seafood	Parmesan Crusted Fish	Lean Cuisine	~~290~~ 300
Seafood	Tortilla Crusted Fish	Lean Cuisine	~~300~~ 310

That's it. At this writing, there are just not that many frozen fish dinners for sale at supermarkets, although new entrees are being introduced continually. If you choose any of the above entrees, you will not use all of the **340 Calories allocated for this meal**. In this case, use the excess 100 or so calories anyway you wish. Splurge on extra dessert or save the calories for another day!

See **Appendix A** on page 197 for our comprehensive list of frozen entrees. Please read the important **Frozen-Food Safety Warning** in **Appendix C** on page 203.

Diet Tip of the Day: **Muscle** is active tissue, fat is not. The more muscle you have, the more calories you burn. Muscle uses a significant number of calories every day for repair and rebuilding, giving your metabolism a boost even when you're resting. So make sure strengthening exercises (like weight lifting) are part of your workout.

Day 66 - Recipe

Pita Pizza

6 pita bread loaves (Joseph's Flax, Oat Bran & Whole Wheat Pita Bread - 8 oz pkg)
¾ cup part-skim shredded mozzarella, divided
1 large red pepper, sliced
1 medium onion, sliced
6 medium mushrooms, sliced
¾ cup tomato sauce, divided
4 tablespoons olive oil

Cook olive oil in large skillet over medium-high heat. Add pepper slices, onion slices and mushroom slices and sauté until they softened.

Toast pita loaves slightly (so they don't get soggy when sauce is applied). Coat one side of pita with tomato sauce. Arrange pepper, onion and mushroom slices on individual pita loaves and sprinkle shredded mozzarella cheese on top.

In oven preheated to 400°F, place pita loaves on baking tin coated with cooking spray. Cook approximately 5 minutes or until cheese melts. Season with salt and pepper to taste.

<u>Serves 3</u>. 430 Calories per serving (Two Pita Pizzas per serving.)

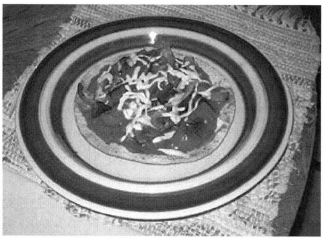

Note only one pita pizza shown. Serving size is <u>two</u> pita pizzas.

Diet Tip of the Day: On a reducing diet, **when you lose – you win**! You win a much better chance for a longer healthier life; you win a sense of well-being; you win a more attractive appearance – and finally you win a feeling of accomplishment.

Chicken Dinner - Out

No recipe today. No cooking today. Have a chicken dinner at your favorite restaurant, but make sure you choose a restaurant where you have a fighting chance to achieve your calorie goal. For your chicken dinner out, your maximum allowable calories (includes appetizer, soup, main course and dessert) are as follows:

- For **1200 Calorie Diet**: 530 Calories
- For **1500 Calorie Diet**: 630 Calories
- For **1800 Calorie Diet**: 630 Calories

Tips for Eating Chicken Out: First, order simple and order skinless white meat only, such as broiled chicken breast with steamed vegetables and brown rice. Tell the waiter you want no sauce, no gravy, nothing added. Then, knowing your calorie objective, and that chicken is about 50 Calories per ounce, most steamed vegetable servings average approximately 50 Calories per cup, and rice is about 100 Calories per ½ cup, decide how much to eat – and take the remainder home. If fresh fruit is not an option, pass on dessert and have the evening snack specified for that day in this diet.

In a restaurant, some nutritionists recommend you eat the low-calorie items on your plate first. Start with the salad, soup and veggies. By the time you get to the chicken and starches you will hopefully be full enough to be content with smaller portions of the higher-calorie choices. (Incidentally, feel free to substitute skinless white meat turkey for chicken.)

Finally, some dieticians advise their dieting clients not to eat out. That's right. They believe eating at home is safer. But our thought is you have to eat out eventually so why not learn how while your resolve is high?

Diet Tip of the Day: When you are eating out, consider **ordering children's portions** or a small sandwich as a way to trim calories and get the size of your meals under control.

Day 68 - Recipe
Pork Medallions in Lime Sauce

1   pound pork tenderloin
⅓   cup all purpose flour
2   tablespoons olive oil
1   tablespoon unsalted butter
½   cup of white wine
¼   cup lime juice
2   stalks celery, chopped
1   medium onion, chopped

Trim away the thin silver skin on the tenderloin and all visible fat. Discard trimmings. Cut tenderloin into ½ to ¾ inch thick medallions. Sprinkle medallions with salt and pepper. Place flour in a shallow dish and coat pork medallions. Warm olive oil in a large skillet over medium-low heat. Working in batches if necessary, cook pork medallions, turning once, until well browned on both sides, about 5 minutes total. (Note internal pork temperature should be 160° F.) Transfer pork to a plate.

Add the wine and lime juice to skillet and bring to boil, scraping up browned bits from bottom of pan with wooden spoon and stirring occasionally, until thickened, about 4 minutes. Remove from heat; stir in butter, chopped celery and onion. Return pork to pan and warm though, turning medallions to coat with sauce.

Serves 4. 450 Calories per serving (pork medallions and sauce only)

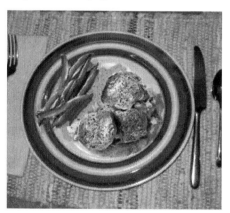

Diet Tip of the Day: Protein and carbohydrates are about 4 Calories per gram (110 Calories per ounce) and fat is 9 Calories per gram (260 Calories per ounce).

Day 69 - Recipe

<u>Healthy Chicken Salad</u>

4   skinless, boneless chicken breast halves, cooked
2   beefsteak tomatoes, cut into large pieces
1   celery heart, chopped
¼   pound roasted red peppers, from jar, chopped
1   small red onion, peeled, halved
10 black olives, halved
1   small bunch basil, leaves only
1½ tablespoons red wine vinegar
3   tablespoons extra-virgin olive oil
¼   pound croutons

Shred cooked chicken and mix with croutons, tomatoes, celery, roasted peppers, red onion, olives and basil in large bowl and season with salt and black pepper. Drizzle with 3 tablespoons extra-virgin olive oil and balsamic vinegar and toss.
<u>Serves 4.</u> 330 Calories per serving

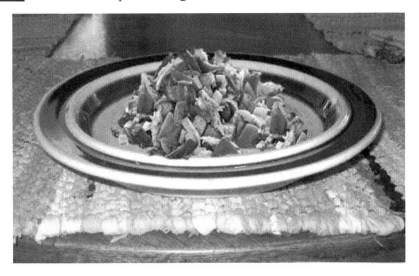

<u>Diet Tip of the Day:</u> In the view of many nutritionists, if you can afford it, buy local and **organic** but you don't have to buy organic across the board because not all organic-labeled products offer added health value.

Day 70 - Recipe

Baked Cod

4 cod fish fillets (4 to 5 ounces each)
2 tablespoons flour
2 tablespoons cornmeal
2 tablespoons minced fresh herbs
2 teaspoons lemon juice
Sprinkle cod with lemon juice. Mix flour, cornmeal and herbs and dust the cod with the cornmeal-herb mixture. Bake in oven at 375 °F for 10 minutes. Add salt and black pepper to taste.
Serves 4. One serving is 230 Calories (cod only).

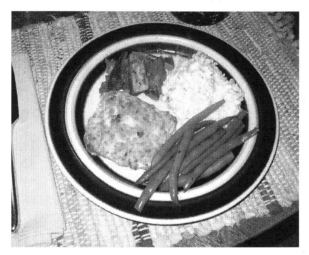

Diet Tip of the Day: It's worth **buying organic** for the "dirty dozen": peaches, strawberries, nectarines, apples, spinach, celery, pears, sweet bell peppers, cherries, potatoes, lettuce, and imported grapes. These fragile fruits and vegetables often require more pesticides to fight off bugs.

Chicken Scaloppini

4   skinless, boneless 6-oz chicken breast halves
2   teaspoons fresh lemon juice
⅓   cup Italian-seasoned breadcrumbs
½   cup fat-free, less-sodium chicken broth
¼   cup dry white wine
4   teaspoons capers
1   tablespoon extra-virgin olive oil

Place each chicken breast half between 2 sheets heavy-duty plastic wrap and pound to about ¼-inch thick using meat mallet. Cut each breast in quarters. Brush chicken with juice, and sprinkle with salt and black pepper. Dredge chicken in breadcrumbs.

Heat a large nonstick skillet coated with cooking spray over medium-high heat. Add chicken to pan; cook 3 minutes on each side or until chicken is done. Remove from pan; keep warm.

Add broth and wine to pan, and cook 30 seconds, stirring constantly. Remove from heat. Stir in capers and olive oil – and serve immediately. **Serves 4**. 260 Calories per serving (chicken only)

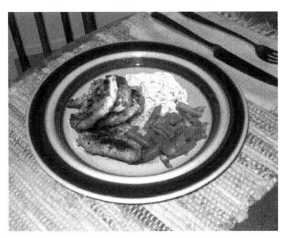

Diet Tip of the Day: Nutritionists define a "**junk food**" as a food that offers little if any essential nutrients – except calories – and when eaten it replaces more important foods.

Day 72 - Recipe

Fish Dinner - Out

No recipe today. No cooking today. Have a fish dinner at your favorite restaurant, but make sure you choose a restaurant where you have a good chance to achieve your calorie goal. For today, your **goal for dinner is a maximum of 595 Calories**. This includes appetizer, soup, main course and dessert.

Tips for Eating Fish Out: The following is almost an exact repeat of the advice given eating out on previous days. First, order simple, such as broiled fish with steamed vegetables and brown rice. Tell the waiter you want no sauce, no gravy, nothing added. Then, knowing your calorie objective, and that fish is about 50 Calories per ounce, most steamed vegetable servings average approximately 50 Calories per cup, and rice is about 100 Calories per ½ cup, decide how much to eat – and take the remainder home. If fresh fruit is not an option, pass on dessert and have the evening snack specified for that day in the diet.

In a restaurant, some nutritionists recommend you eat the low-calorie items on your plate first. Start with the salad, soup and veggies. By the time you get to the fish and starches you will hopefully be full enough to be content with smaller portions of the higher-calorie choices.

Diet Tip of the Day: In the U.S., we consume more than 100 pounds of **sugar** per year per person, totaling an unhealthy, nutritionally empty, 500 Calories per day. This large intake of sugar leads to obvious ills, such as obesity and tooth decay.

Day 73 - Recipe

Pasta Pomodoro

Pasta Pomodoro (Italian for pasta with tomatoes) is typically prepared with angel hair pasta, olive oil, fresh tomatoes, and fresh basil. It's light, delicious and easy to make.

¾ pound angel hair pasta
1½ pints cherry tomatoes (about 45), halved
8   fresh basil leaves, chopped
4   cloves garlic, minced
2   tablespoons olive oil
4   Tbsp grated parmesan cheese

Cook angel hair pasta per package directions. Over medium heat, sauté the garlic in olive oil until it just starts to turn golden. Add tomatoes and cook for about 10 minutes, or until they just start to release juices. Turn off the heat and stir basil into the sauce. Over the cooked pasta, spoon the tomato sauce with a little of the pasta water and garnish with more basil and grated cheese.

Serves 4. 420 Calories per serving

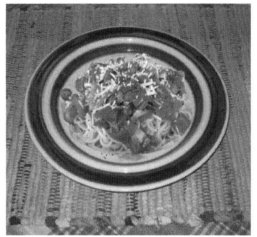

Above prepared with mix of cherry and plum tomatoes.

Diet Tip of the Day: Thinking about using **honey** rather than sugar? Honey has about 21 calories per teaspoon while sugar has 15. And the vitamin and mineral content of honey is very low.

Day 74 - Recipe

Frozen Chicken Dinner

No recipe today. No cooking today. Another day off! There are plenty of frozen chicken choices in your local supermarket. Here are some reasonably good selections:

Poultry	Crustless Chicken Pot Pie	Smart Ones	~~200~~ 190
Poultry	Buffalo Style Chicken	Lean Cuisine	~~200~~ 190
Poultry	Home Style Chicken & Potatoes	Healthy Choice	200
Poultry	Honey Balsamic Chicken	Healthy Choice	210
Poultry	Sesame Stir Fry with Chicken	Lean Cuisine	280
Poultry	Roasted Turkey Breast	Lean Cuisine	~~280~~ 290
Poultry	Apple Cranberry Chicken	Lean Cuisine	280
Poultry	Chicken Fettuccini Alfredo	Healthy Choice	280
Poultry	Grilled Chicken Marinara	Healthy Choice	280
Poultry	Sweet & Spicy Orange Chicken	Healthy Choice	280
Poultry	Chicken Parmesan	Smart Ones	280
Poultry	Turkey Breast with Stuffing	Smart Ones	280

If you choose the first four meals above, you will fall far short of the **300 Calories allocated for today's frozen meal.** In this case, use the remaining 100 or so calories anyway you wish. Splurge on extra dessert or save the calories for another day.

See **Appendix A** on page 197 for our comprehensive list of frozen entrees. Please read the important **Frozen-Food Safety Warning** in **Appendix C** on page 203.

<u>Diet Tip of the Day:</u> Many health care professionals think that eating a healthy **vegetarian diet** is one of the best things you can do for your short-term and long-term health. But a vegetarian diet must be carefully planned.

Szechuan Noodles and Pork

8   ounces linguine pasta
1   cup chicken broth
2   tablespoon light soy sauce
8   ounces ground pork (lean)
¼   teaspoon red pepper flakes
6   scallions, cut in ½-inch pieces
1   large carrot, shredded
1   tablespoon each minced garlic and ginger
1½ tablespoons creamy peanut butter

Cook linguine per package directions. Mix broth and soy sauce in a measuring cup.

Cook ground pork and red pepper flakes in large non-stick skillet over medium-high heat for about 5 minutes. Make sure pork is browned and no longer pink. Add scallions, carrot, garlic and ginger; cook additional 3 minutes. Stir broth mixture and peanut butter into pork. Cook until peanut butter melts and is blended.

Drain linguine, add to skillet and toss to evenly coat with sauce. (Use some cooking water if needed to keep mixture creamy.) Garnish with cilantro.

Serves 4. 440 Calories per serving.

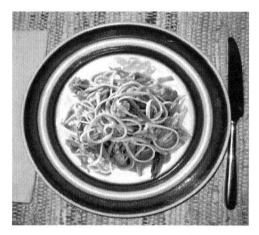

Diet Tip of the Day: Studies have shown **vegetarian** diets significantly lower the risk of colon cancer, heart disease, high blood pressure and other diseases.

Day 76 - Recipe
Gary & Sue's Grilled Scallops

We were invited by our good friends, Gary and Sue, for dinner. They prepared a simple, but nutritious low-calorie meal – which featured scallops. (Scallops are a very low calorie food – expensive but great when you're on a diet.) The photo below is our version of the main course they served that night.

1½   pounds sea scallops
3   medium tomatoes, sliced, divided
4   ears of corn
2   tablespoons olive oil, divided
1   tablespoon balsamic vinegar, divided

Place scallops in a shallow bowl. Add olive oil and vinegar and toss to coat. Grill scallops on medium-hot fire. Turn after two minutes or when first side turns opaque. Grill until second side turns opaque – about another 2 minutes. Don't overcook but test a scallop by cutting to make sure it's cooked through. Salt and black pepper to taste.

Serves 4. The food pictured on the plate below totals about 360 Calories.

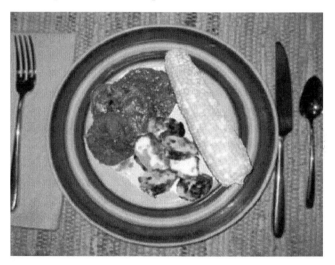

Diet Tip of the Day: When you eat fiber, it simply passes straight through, untouched by but aiding your digestive system. **Zero calories absorbed!**

Day 77 - Recipe
Chicken with Peppers and Rice

4 boneless, skinless chicken breast halves (about 1 lb)
1 red bell pepper, sliced
1 green bell pepper, sliced
1 yellow bell pepper, sliced
1 medium onion, sliced
1 ounce package of herb, garlic dip and soup mix
2 tablespoons olive oil
¾ cup wild rice, brown rice and wheat-berry mix.

Prepare wild rice per package directions. Cut chicken into 2 to 3-inch pieces. Place vegetables and chicken in re-sealable plastic bag. Add seasoning blend and olive oil. Seal bag and refrigerate for about two hours. Preheat oven to 400°F. Place chicken and peppers in foil-lined baking pan. (Discard any remaining liquid in bag.) Bake 30 to 40 minutes, or until chicken is done. Broil an additional 2 to 3 minutes to brown chicken (optional).

<u>Serves 4</u>. 290 Calories per serving (Chicken, peppers and wild rice)

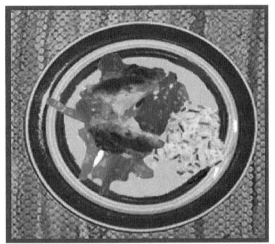

Chicken was browned too much but was still quite tasty!

<u>Diet Tip of the Day:</u> Most Americans consume too much sodium (salt). The U.S. Department of Agriculture Dietary Guidelines recommend that healthy adults **limit sodium intake to 2400 mg per day**. (One teaspoon of salt contains about 2300 mg of sodium.)

Day 78 - Recipe
Trout with Lemon &Capers

4   trout fillets (4-oz each), skin attached
3   tablespoons unsalted butter, divided
2   tablespoons olive oil
2   tablespoons lemon juice
4   teaspoons chopped parsley
1   teaspoon capers
2   small lemons peeled and segmented

Score 2 crosswise slits (skin deep only) into each trout fillet using sharp knife. Turn the fillets over and season flesh with the salt and pepper.

Heat 1 tablespoon butter and the olive oil in a large nonstick skillet over medium-high heat. Place the fillets in the nonstick skillet, skin side up, and cook until golden brown, about 3 minutes. Turn and continue until cooked through and the skin begins to crisp around edges, about 2 more minutes. Transfer fillets to serving dish and keep warm.

Add the remaining 2 tablespoons butter to the hot skillet and cook until just brown. Stir in the lemon juice, parsley, capers, and lemon segments. Pour sauce over fillets and serve.

Serves 4. 340 Calories per serving (trout and sauce only)

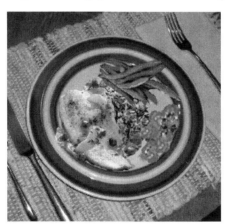

Diet Tip of the Day: Nearly every animal food, including dairy products, eggs, meat, poultry and fish are **complete proteins** because they contain all eight-essential amino acids. Soy is the only plant-based food that has all eight essential-amino acids.

Day 79 - Recipe

Chinese Dinner - Out

No recipe today. No cooking today. Have a Chinese dinner at your favorite restaurant, but make sure you choose a restaurant where you have a reasonable chance to achieve your calorie goal. For today, **your goal for dinner is a maximum of 640 Calories**. This includes any appetizer, soup, main course and any dessert.

Tips for Eating Chinese: You can consume a lot of calories in a Chinese restaurant – if you order carelessly. For example a typical portion of General Tso's chicken is loaded with about 1,000 Calories, then add another 200 Calories for a cup of rice.

First rule, order simple. Look for an entree with lots of vegetables, some fish or chicken and brown rice. Tell the waiter you want your food steamed with any sauce on the side. (This is not only a low-calorie way of eating Chinese food but is also the most nutritious way to eat Chinese food.)

Then, knowing your 640 Calorie objective, and that chicken and fish are about 50 Calories per ounce, most steamed vegetable servings average approximately 50 Calories per cup, and rice is about 200 Calories per cup, decide how much of the meal you can eat – and take the remainder home. (Note that you will be eating half a serving of left over Chinese food for lunch tomorrow.) To stay within your maximum allowable calorie total, you should pass on dessert and have the evening snack specified for that day in the diet.

Incidentally, although Chinese is specified, feel free to substitute Thai food, Vietnamese, Indian, Middle Eastern, or any other favorite ethnic food. Just make sure you don't exceed the maximum allowable 640 calories for this meal.

Diet Tip of the Day: Know your **daily caloric allowance** whether you are trying to maintain your weight or are on a reducing diet. (See "*Weight Control - U.S. Edition*" a NoPaperPress eBook where you can determine your daily caloric allowance using unique Weight Maintenance tables.)

Day 80 - Recipe

Vegetable Chili

1 tablespoon olive oil
2 medium carrots, cut into ½-inch pieces
2 medium parsnips, cut into ½-inch pieces
1 medium onion, chopped
2 cans (15-ounces each) red kidney beans, drained
4 teaspoons chili powder
1 can (28-ounce) whole tomatoes in juice
¼ cup fresh cilantro leaves, chopped

In saucepot, heat olive oil on medium-high. Add carrots, parsnips, chopped onion, and cook 6 to 8 minutes or until all vegetables are tender and beginning to brown, stirring occasionally.

Meanwhile, on large plate, mash 1 cup drained beans. Stir chili powder into vegetables in saucepot; cook 1 minute, stirring. Add canned tomatoes with their juice, whole and mashed beans, and 2 cups water. Heat to boiling on high, breaking up tomatoes with spoon. Reduce heat to medium and cook, uncovered for 10 minutes, stirring occasionally. Finally, stir in cilantro and serve.

Serves 4. 360 Calories per serving

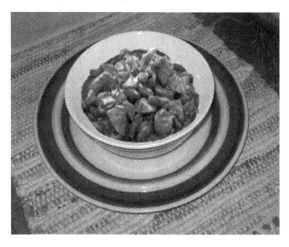

Diet Tip of the Day: **Carbohydrates** provide your body with its basic fuel, the energy your cells need to survive, as well as essential vitamins and minerals, fiber, and other beneficial compounds that promote good health.

Day 81 - Recipe
Frozen-Meat Dinner

No recipe today. No cooking today. Another day off! That's it. At this writing, there are just not that many frozen meat dinners for sale at supermarkets, although new entrees are being introduced continually. Here are some reasonably good frozen-meat dinners:

Meat	Steak Portobella	Lean Cuisine	160
Meat	Asian Style Beef & Broccoli	Smart Ones	~~160~~ 170
Meat	Beef Merlot	Healthy Choice	180
Meat	Home style Beef Pot Roast	Smart Ones	180
Meat	Salisbury Steak with Mac & Cheese	Lean Cuisine	~~270~~ 290
Pasta	Pasta with Swedish Meatballs	Smart Ones	~~280~~ 290
Meat	Classic Meat Loaf	Healthy Choice	300

If you choose any of the above entrees, you will fall short of the **300 Calories allocated for this day**. In this case, use the remaining calories anyway you wish. Indulge on extra dessert or save the calories for another day.

See **Appendix A** on page 197 for our comprehensive list of frozen entrees. Please read the important **Frozen-Food Safety Warning** in **Appendix C** on page 203.

Diet Tip of the Day: Keep low-calorie **lean sandwich fixings on hand** (whole-wheat bread, sliced turkey, reduced-fat cheese, lettuce, tomatoes and mustard).

Day 82 - Recipe

Chinese Chicken Salad

4 skinless, boneless chicken breast halves (½ lb total)
1 cup carrots, sliced
1 cup red bell peppers, sliced
4 green onions, diced
1 cup edamame beans, cooked and shelled
1 cup chow mien noodles
2 hearts romaine lettuce
4 cups mesclun mix or spring mix

<u>Chinese salad dressing</u>: In a jar with a tight-fitting lid combine 2 tsp garlic powder, 1 tsp dried parsley, 1 tsp dried basil, 1 tsp honey, 2 tsp soy sauce, 4 tsp sesame oil, 2 tsp Sriracha (Chinese hot sauce – optional), 4 tsp Dijon mustard, 4 tbsp olive oil, 4 tbsp rice wine vinegar and a dash of black pepper. Shake well and set aside.

Grill chicken breast halves and then cut them into small pieces.

In a bowl, combine romaine lettuce, mesclun mix lettuces (or spring mix), carrots, red bell pepper, green onions and edamame. Add the dressing and toss. Add chow mien noodles and chicken and toss again.

Serves 4. 440 Calories per serving

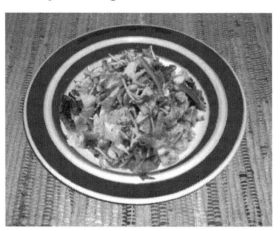

Diet Tip of the Day: Do not eat foods containing partially-hydrogenated vegetable oil because they are high in **trans fats**. This includes commercially prepared baked goods, snack foods, and processed foods, including most fast foods.

Day 83 - Recipe

Hearty Lentil Stew

½ cup chopped onion
2 garlic cloves, minced
1 tablespoon vegetable oil
1 cup lentils, rinsed
4 tsp vegetable or chicken bouillon granules
3 tsp Worcestershire sauce
1 bay leaf
1 cup chopped carrots
14.5-ounce can diced tomatoes with liquid
10-oz package frozen chopped spinach, thawed
1 Tbsp red wine vinegar

In a large saucepan, sauté onion and garlic in oil until tender. Add 5 cups of water, lentils, bouillon, Worcestershire sauce, ½ teaspoon salt, ¼ teaspoon black pepper and the bay leaf. Bring to a boil. Reduce heat; cover and simmer for 20 minutes.

Add the carrots, tomatoes and spinach; return to a boil. Reduce heat; cover and simmer additional 15 to 20 minutes, or until lentils are tender. Stir in vinegar and serve.

Serves 4. 260 Calories per serving

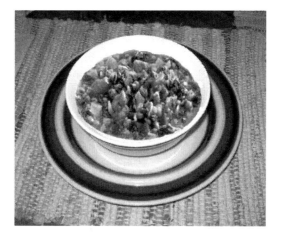

Diet Tip of the Day: Monounsaturated fats "**good fats**" are derived from plant sources, such as vegetable oils, nuts, and seeds. This type of fat is found in high concentrations in canola, olive and peanut oils.

Day 84 - Recipe

Turkey Burger

1¼ pounds ground turkey
1   tablespoon Worcestershire sauce
1   tablespoon chipotle mustard
1   tablespoon olive oil for brushing
4   seeded hamburger rolls

Lightly mix together the ground turkey, Worcestershire sauce, mustard, salt and black pepper. Form into 4 patties and brush each side lightly with olive oil.

Heat grill to medium-high. Place patties on grill and cook for 3 to 4 minutes each side for medium-well done. Salt and pepper to taste.
Serves 4. 355 Calories per serving (turkey burger only)

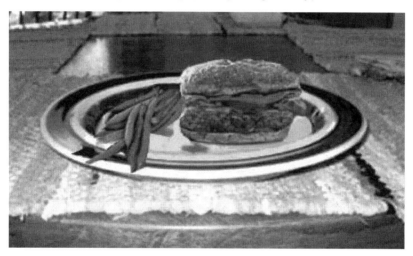

Diet Tip of the Day: Consistently **choose healthy foods**, avoid harmful foods and large portions and exercise regularly. Nothing else will control your weight over the long haul.

Day 85 - Recipe
Carrie's Low-Cal Meat Loaf

½ pound ground white meat turkey
½ pound ground beef (about 90% lean)
1 large egg
½ cup skim milk
¼ cup bread crumbs
¼ cup ketchup
¼ cup chopped carrots
¼ cup chopped onion

In a medium bowl, combine all ingredients. Add salt and pepper to taste. Mix until blended and form into a loaf. Place loaf into oven preheated to 350 °F. Bake until an instant-read thermometer inserted in the center of the loaf reads 160 °F. This should take about one hour.

Shown below is meat loaf, acorn squash (baked with 1 teaspoon of maple syrup). Also shown is steamed spinach drizzled with extra-virgin olive oil. **Serves 5**. About 290 Calories per serving (for meat loaf only). Note that half a serving of left over meat loaf is to be eaten for lunch on Day 87.

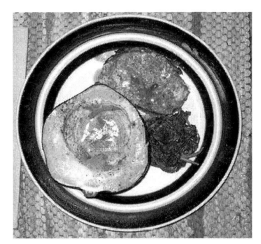

Diet Tip of the Day: Your **body weight fluctuates** two to three pounds daily. Your body weight is lowest before breakfast and highest in the evening before you retire.

Day 86 - Recipe

Tuna & Bean Salad

1   tuna steak, about 2 inches thick (14 ounces)
2   tablespoons extra-virgin olive oil
1   tablespoon lemon juice
1   garlic clove, crushed
1   tablespoon Dijon mustard
1   15-ounce can cannellini beans, drained
1   small red onion, thinly sliced
2   red peppers, seeded and thinly sliced
½   cucumber, halved lengthwise and thinly sliced
6   cups watercress

Heat a ridged grill pan coated with cooking spray over medium-high heat. Season tuna steak on both sides with coarsely ground black pepper. Cook the tuna 4 minutes on each side - the outside should be browned and the center light pink. Be careful not to overcook. Remove from the pan and set aside.

Mix together the oil, lemon juice, garlic, and mustard in a salad bowl. Season with salt and pepper to taste. Add the cannellini beans, onion, peppers, cucumber and watercress. Toss gently to mix. Cut tuna into ½-inch thick slices. Arrange on top of salad and serve with lemon wedges. **Serves 4**. 355 Calories per serving

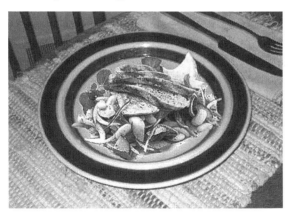

Diet Tip of the Day: In the United States, for a food to be labeled "**whole grain**" it must contain more than 51 percent whole grain by weight.

Day 87 - Recipe

Pasta Primavera

¾ pound penne pasta
2 cups broccoli florets
1 red bell pepper, sliced
1 carrot, cut to 1-inch sticks
½ cup frozen green peas & ½ cup frozen sweet corn
1 small onion, chopped
1 tablespoon minced garlic
3 tablespoons olive oil
1 teaspoon fresh basil, chopped

Cook penne pasta per package directions. Drain and place pasta in a bowl.
Pre-cook the carrot and broccoli florets.

In a large heavy skillet, heat the olive oil and sauté onion and garlic until
lightly golden. Add vegetables and sauté until the peppers are soft.
Combine sautéed vegetables in the bowl with the pasta. Toss well. Garnish
with chopped basil, season to taste, and top with freshly grated Parmesan
cheese.

Serves 4. 460 Calories per serving

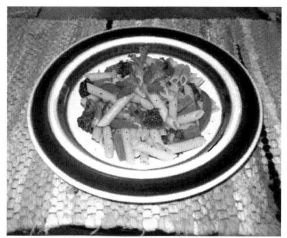

Photo taken before grated cheese was added.

Diet Tip of the Day: When possible, **select fresh and natural foods** and
whole-grain products. Avoid chemical preservatives and additives,
artificial and imitation foods, refined and processed foods, and foods that
are comprised of "nutritionally-empty calories."

Day 88 - Recipe
Frozen Chicken Dinner

No recipe today. No cooking today. Another day off! There are plenty of frozen chicken choices in your local supermarket. Here are some reasonably good selections:

Poultry	Crustless Chicken Pot Pie	Smart Ones	~~200~~ 190
Poultry	Buffalo Style Chicken	Lean Cuisine	~~200~~ 190
Poultry	Home Style Chicken & Potatoes	Healthy Choice	200
Poultry	Honey Balsamic Chicken	Healthy Choice	210
Poultry	Sesame Stir Fry with Chicken	Lean Cuisine	280
Poultry	Roasted Turkey Breast	Lean Cuisine	~~280~~ 290
Poultry	Apple Cranberry Chicken	Lean Cuisine	280
Poultry	Chicken Fettuccini Alfredo	Healthy Choice	280
Poultry	Grilled Chicken Marinara	Healthy Choice	280
Poultry	Sweet & Spicy Orange Chicken	Healthy Choice	280
Poultry	Chicken Parmesan	Smart Ones	280
Poultry	Turkey Breast with Stuffing	Smart Ones	280

If you choose the first four meals above, you will fall far short of the **300 Calories allocated for today's frozen meal.** In this case, use the remaining 100 or so calories anyway you wish. Splurge on extra dessert or save the calories for another day.

See **Appendix A** on page 197 for our comprehensive list of frozen entrees. Please read the important **Frozen-Food Safety Warning** in **Appendix C** on page 203.

Diet Tip of the Day: Understand that the only **sure way to slim down for keeps** is to eat less and exercise more. There are no safe short cuts or miracle methods for taking off weight.

Day 89 - Recipe

Fish Stew

1	pound shrimp, peeled and de-veined
¾	pound skinless flounder fillet, cut into strips
1	pound new baby potatoes, halved
2	peppers (red and yellow) sliced into strips
1	onion, halved and sliced
4	ounces white wine
2	cups vegetable stock
2	cloves garlic, crushed
1	small bunch basil, shredded
1½	tablespoons olive oil

In a large pot, sauté garlic, onion and peppers in olive oil until they are completely softened. Stir in wine, vegetable stock and potatoes. Simmer until potatoes are tender.

Add the shrimp and flounder and cook for additional 4 minutes. Stir in basil and serve.

Serves 4. 300 Calories per serving

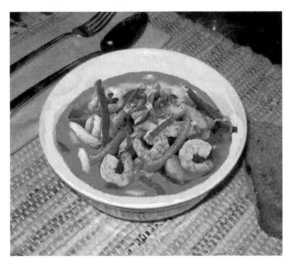

Diet Tip of the Day: All **fish** are relatively low-calorie foods and are good sources of protein and fat-soluble vitamins A and D.

Day 90 - Recipe
Veal with Mushrooms & Tomato

½ pound spaghetti
¾ pound veal cutlets
8 ounces sliced mushrooms
2 tablespoon olive oil, divided
2 tablespoons flour
3 green onions, small, sliced
½ cup chicken broth
14.5-ounce can diced tomatoes

Pound veal to about ¼-inch thickness. Rinse, pat dry and cut into 2-inch pieces. Heat 1 tablespoon olive oil in large nonstick skillet over medium heat. Add mushrooms and cook, stirring, until lightly browned. Remove and set aside.

Season veal with salt and pepper and coat lightly with flour. Add remaining olive oil to skillet and cook veal over medium heat for about 2 minutes on each side, or until browned. Add the green onions and cook for 1 minute longer. Add chicken broth and cook, uncovered, for 5 minutes. Add tomatoes; cover and simmer for 3 to 5 minutes. Serve over spaghetti cooked per package directions.

Serves 4. 520 Calories per serving (includes spaghetti)

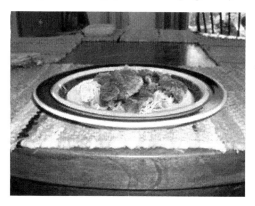

Diet Tip of the Day: Successful weight loss and subsequent weight maintenance **requires knowledge, desire and discipline**. Avoid the latest fad diets. Instead, take the time to develop a true understanding of weight control and then change your eating and activity habits accordingly.

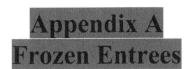

Appendix A
Frozen Entrees

Appendix D lists three popular brands of frozen entrées: Healthy Choice, Lean Cuisine and Smart Ones. Note that each brand is color coded. The listing is further divided by entrée type: Poultry entrées, Meat entrées, Seafood entrées, Pasta entrées, Pizza and Other entrées. The entire table is arranged from the lowest to highest in calories. Note that the listed frozen entrées were available in most super markets as of 07/21/2020.

Entrée Type	Name	Brand	Calories
Poultry	Tomato Basil Chicken & Spinach	Smart Ones	160
Meat	Steak Portobella	Lean Cuisine	160
Meat	Asian Style Beef & Broccoli	Smart Ones	~~160~~ 170
Poultry	Herb Roasted Chicken	Lean Cuisine	170
Poultry	Slow Roasted Turkey Breast	Smart Ones	170
Poultry	Grilled Chicken Marsala	Healthy Choice	180
Poultry	Creamy Basil Chicken w Broccoli	Smart Ones	~~180~~ 170
Poultry	Garlic Chicken Rolls	Lean Cuisine	180
Meat	Beef Merlot	Healthy Choice	180
Meat	Homestyle Beef Pot Roast	Smart Ones	180
Poultry	Roasted Turkey & Vegetables	Lean Cuisine	190
Poultry	Chicken & Broccoli Alfredo	Healthy Choice	190
Poultry	Chicken & Vegetable Stir Fry	Healthy Choice	190
Other	Broccoli & Cheddar Roast Potato	Smart Ones	190
Poultry	Home Style Chicken & Potatoes	Healthy Choice	200
Poultry	Crustless Chicken Pot Pie	Smart Ones	~~200~~ 190
Poultry	Buffalo Style Chicken	Lean Cuisine	~~200~~ 190
Pasta	Angel Hair Marinara	Smart Ones	200
Poultry	Salisbury Steak	Smart Ones	200
Meat	Roast Beef & Mashed Potatoes	Smart Ones	~~220~~ 200
Pasta	Primavera Pasta	Smart Ones	210
Poultry	Honey Balsamic Chicken	Healthy Choice	210

Pasta	Ravioli Florentine	Smart Ones	210
Poultry	Cajun Style Chicken & Shrimp	Healthy Choice	220
Pasta	Cheese Ravioli Mushroom Sauce	Smart Ones	230
Poultry	Ranchero Chicken Wrap	Smart Ones	230
Poultry	Lemon Herb Chicken Picante	Smart Ones	230
Pasta	Cheese Ravioli Mushroom Sauce	Smart Ones	230
Meat	Meat Loaf with Mashed Potatoes	Lean Cuisine	~~230~~ 240
Seafood	Shrimp Alfredo	Lean Cuisine	~~230~~ 240
Poultry	Chicken Margherita	Smart Ones	~~220~~ 240
Poultry	Grilled Chicken Caesar	Lean Cuisine	240
Poultry	Honey Glazed Turkey & Potatoes	Healthy Choice	240
Pasta	Spicy Penne Arrabbiata	Lean Cuisine	240
Pasta	Four Cheese Cannelloni	Lean Cuisine	~~240~~ 250
Poultry	Creamy Basil Chicken w Tortellini	Lean Cuisine	~~240~~ 250
Pasta	Cheese Ravioli	Lean Cuisine	250
Pasta	Vermont Cheddar Mac & Cheese	Lean Cuisine	250
Pasta	Fettuccini Alfredo	Smart Ones	250
Poultry	Oriental Chicken	Smart Ones	250
Poultry	Fiesta Grilled Chicken	Lean Cuisine	250
Pasta	Chicken Linguini Red Pepper	Healthy Choice	250
Poultry	Golden Roasted Turkey Breast	Healthy Choice	250
Poultry	Chicken Mesquite	Smart Ones	250
Poultry	Chicken Oriental	Smart Ones	250
Poultry	Orange Sesame Chicken	Smart Ones	250
Poultry	Baked Chicken	Lean Cuisine	~~250~~ 260
Poultry	Teriyaki Chicken & Vegetables	Smart Ones	~~250~~ 260
Seafood	Tuna Noodle Casserole	Smart Ones	~~250~~ 270
Pasta	Spaghetti with Meatballs	Lean Cuisine	260
Poultry	Creamy Chicken & Noodles	Healthy Choice	260
Meat	Barbecue Steak w Red Potatoes	Healthy Choice	260
Pasta	Tortellini Primavera Parmesan	Healthy Choice	260
Pasta	Sesame Noodles with Vegetables	Smart Ones	~~260~~ 280

Pasta	Creamy Rigatoni w Chicken	Smart Ones	260
Pasta	Macaroni & Cheese	Smart Ones	260
Pasta	Butternut Squash Ravioli	Lean Cuisine	260
Other	Santa Fe Rice & Beans	Smart Ones	260
Other	Coconut Chickpea Curry	Lean Cuisine	260
Poultry	Glazed Turkey Tenderloins	Lean Cuisine	270
Poultry	Kung Pao Chicken	Healthy Choice	270
Poultry	Chicken Margherita w Balsamic	Healthy Choice	270
Poultry	Chicken Strips & Sweet Potatoes	Smart Ones	270
Pasta	Spaghetti with Meat Sauce	Smart Ones	~~270~~ 280
Meat	Salisbury Steak with Mac & Cheese	Lean Cuisine	~~270~~ 290
Pasta	Penne Rosa	Lean Cuisine	270
Poultry	Turkey Breast & Stuffing	Smart Ones	~~270~~ 280
Pasta	Classic Macaroni & Beef	Lean Cuisine	270
Pasta	Mushroom Mezzaluna Ravioli	Lean Cuisine	270
Pasta	Pasta with Swedish Meatballs	Smart Ones	~~280~~ 290
Other	Asian Pot Stickers	Lean Cuisine	280
Poultry	Sesame Stir Fry with Chicken	Lean Cuisine	280
Poultry	Roasted Turkey Breast	Lean Cuisine	~~280~~ 290
Poultry	Apple Cranberry Chicken	Lean Cuisine	280
Poultry	Chicken Fettuccini Alfredo	Healthy Choice	280
Poultry	Grilled Chicken Marinara	Healthy Choice	280
Poultry	Sweet & Spicy Orange Chicken	Healthy Choice	280
Poultry	Chicken Parmesan	Smart Ones	280
Poultry	Turkey Breast with Stuffing	Smart Ones	280
Meat	Beef & Broccoli	Healthy Choice	280
Meat	Meatball Marinara	Healthy Choice	280
Meat	Beef Teriyaki	Healthy Choice	280
Pasta	Spinach Artichoke Ravioli	Lean Cuisine	280
Other	Vegetable Fried Rice	Smart Ones	280
Pasta	Spinach Artichoke Ravioli	Lean Cuisine	280
Pasta	Linguini with Ricotta & Spinach	Lean Cuisine	280

Poultry	Chicken Fettuccini	Lean Cuisine	~~290~~ 280
Pasta	Spaghetti & Meatballs	Healthy Choice	280
Pasta	Spaghetti with Meat Sauce	Smart Ones	280
Other	Vegetable Fried Rice	Smart Ones	280
Other	Asian Pot Stickers	Lean Cuisine	280
Poultry	Chicken with Almonds	Lean Cuisine	290
Poultry	Chicken with Peanut Sauce	Lean Cuisine	290
Seafood	Shrimp & Angel Hair Pasta	Lean Cuisine	~~280~~ 290
Poultry	Grilled Chicken Pesto w Veggies	Healthy Choice	290
Poultry	General Tso's Spicy Chicken	Healthy Choice	290
Poultry	Pineapple Chicken	Healthy Choice	290
Poultry	Chicken Enchiladas Suiza	Smart Ones	290
Meat	Swedish Meatballs	Lean Cuisine	290
Seafood	Lemon Pepper Fish	Healthy Choice	290
Pasta	Pasta with Swedish Meatballs	Smart Ones	290
Other	Santa Fe Rice & Beans	Smart Ones	290
Pizza	Thin Crust Cheese Pizza	Smart Ones	290
Seafood	Parmesan Crusted Fish	Lean Cuisine	~~290~~ 300
Pasta	Santa Fe-Style Rice & Beans	Lean Cuisine	~~280~~ 300
Poultry	Roasted Turkey & Vegetables	Lean Cuisine	~~290~~ 300
Poultry	Sweet & Sour Chicken	Lean Cuisine	300
Poultry	Crustless Chicken Pot Pie	Healthy Choice	300
Poultry	Sweet Sesame Chicken	Healthy Choice	300
Poultry	Chicken Fettuccini	Smart Ones	300
Poultry	General Tso's Chicken	Smart Ones	300
Meat	Classic Meat Loaf	Healthy Choice	300
Seafood	Tortilla Crusted Fish	Lean Cuisine	~~300~~ 310
Pasta	Tuscan-Style Vegetable Lasagna	Lean Cuisine	~~300~~ 310
Pasta	Tortellini with Red Pepper Sauce	Lean Cuisine	300
Pasta	Broccoli Cheddar Rotini	Lean Cuisine	300
Pasta	Three Cheese Ziti Marinara	Smart Ones	300
Pasta	Lasagna Florentine	Smart Ones	~~310~~ 300

Seafood	Tortilla Crusted Fish	Lean Cuisine	~~300~~ 310
Pasta	Tuscan-Style Vegetable Lasagna	Lean Cuisine	~~300~~ 310
Poultry	Chicken Fried Rice	Lean Cuisine	~~300~~ 310
Poultry	Orange Chicken	Lean Cuisine	310
Poultry	Chicken Tikka Masala	Lean Cuisine	310
Poultry	Chicken Strips & Fries	Smart Ones	310
Poultry	Chicken Teriyaki	Lean Cuisine	310
Pizza	Thin Crust Pepperoni Pizza	Smart Ones	310
Pasta	Three Cheese Macaroni	Smart Ones	310
Pizza	French Bread Pepperoni Pizza	Lean Cuisine	310
Poultry	Chicken Spinach Mushroom Panini	Lean Cuisine	~~350~~ 310
Other	Spicy Beef & Bean Enchilada	Lean Cuisine	310
Poultry	Chicken Fried Rice	Healthy Choice	320
Meat	Sweet & Spicy Korean Beef	Lean Cuisine	320
Pizza	Farmers Market Pizza	Lean Cuisine	320
Pizza	Margherita Pizza	Lean Cuisine	320
Poultry	Chicken Carbonara	Lean Cuisine	330
Poultry	Mango Chicken w Coconut Rice	Lean Cuisine	330
Poultry	Country Fried Chicken	Healthy Choice	330
Other	Cheese & Fire-Roasted Tamale	Lean Cuisine	330
Poultry	Chicken Club Panini	Lean Cuisine	~~350~~ 340
Meat	Philly Style Steak & Cheese Panini	Lean Cuisine	~~330~~ 350
Poultry	Chicken Parmigiana	Healthy Choice	360
Poultry	Chicken Pecan	Lean Cuisine	~~320~~ 370
Poultry	Sweet & Sour Chicken	Healthy Choice	390
Pizza	Supreme Pizza	Lean Cuisine	~~330~~ 390

Appendix B: Soup Selections

When the Daily Meal Plan menu specifies soup have only one serving (8 ounces) unless stated otherwise. Note that the listed soups were available in most supermarkets as of 07/21/2020. *These are a canned soup selections.

Soup Description	Calories
Healthy Choice Chicken with Rice	90
Campbell's Tomato	100
Healthy Choice Country Vegetable	100
Progresso Minestrone*	110
Progresso Chickarina*	110
Progresso Italian-Style Wedding*	120
Campbell's Home-Style Light Chicken Corn Chowder*	120
Campbell's Home-Style Chicken Noodle	130
Campbell's Home-Style Butter Nut Squash*	130
Campbell's Healthy Request Vegetable Beef	140
Progresso Lentil*	140
Progresso Green Split Pea*	150
Campbell's Slow Kettle New England Clam Chowder	160
Progresso Macaroni and Bean*	160
Progresso New England Clam Chowder*	170
Progresso Lasagna-Style*	170
Progresso Broccoli Cheese with Bacon*	180
As an alternative, have 2 servings of 90 Calorie soup	180
Campbell's Chunky Classic Chicken Noodle	190
Amy's Rustic Italian Vegetable*	190
Campbell's Chunky Beef n Cheese*	200
Amy's French Country Vegetable*	210
Campbell's Chunky Sirloin Burger + Vegetables	220
Enjoy two servings of a 110 or 120 Calorie soup	230
Enjoy two servings of a 120 Calorie soup	240

Increasingly, food giants like ConAgra, Nestlé and others that supply Americans with processed foods concede that they cannot ensure the safety of their food products. Frozen foods pose a particularly serious safety problem because unsuspecting consumers buy frozen foods for their convenience and incorrectly believe that cooking frozen foods is a matter of taste – not safety. Still the food industry says that extensive outbreaks of food-borne illness are rare, even though it is well-known that most of the millions of cases of food-borne illness every year go unreported or are not traced to the source. For example, each year approximately 40,000 cases of salmonella poisoning are reported in the United States – but perhaps as many as one million cases go unreported. (Salmonella is a type of bacteria most often found in poultry, eggs, unprocessed milk, meat and water.) Recently salmonella pathogens in some frozen meals have sickened thousands of people.

How could this happen? First, the supply chain for ingredients in processed foods – from flour to fruits and vegetables to flavorings – is becoming more complex and global in the drive to keep food costs down. As a result, government and industry officials concede that almost every food ingredient is now a potential carrier of pathogens. A further complication is that a large number of food companies subcontract processing work to save money and don't require suppliers to test for pathogens. In fact, companies often don't even know who is supplying their ingredients.

In addition, many frozen-food manufacturers have stopped cooking their products at high temperatures, a tactic they call the "kill step," which is intended to eliminate any lingering microbes. Frequently this process step turns some of the frozen food ingredients into mush. So, instead the "kill step" has been shifted to consumers. For example, ConAgra has added food safety instructions to its frozen meals, including the Healthy Choice brand. A typical "frozen-food safety" instruction offers this guidance: "Internal temperature needs to reach 165°F as measured by a food thermometer in several spots."

Moreover, General Mills, now advises consumers to avoid microwaves altogether and cook their frozen pizzas only in a conventional oven. **Bottom line**: To be safe, always cook frozen foods so that the internal temperature reaches 165°F as measured by a good food.

NoPaperPress eBooks and Paperbacks

100-Day Super Diet-1200 Cal*
100-Day Super Diet-1500 Cal*
100-Day No-Cooking Diet-1200 Cal*
100-Day No-Cooking Diet-1500 Cal*
90-Day Smart Diet-1200 Cal*
90-Day Smart Diet-1500 Cal*
90-Day No-Cooking Diet - 1200 Cal*
90-Day No-Cooking Diet - 1500 Cal*
90-Day Perfect Diet - 1200 Cal*
90-Day Perfect Diet - 1500 Cal*
60-Day Perfect Diet-1200 Cal*
60-Day Perfect Diet-1500 Cal*
50-Day Flex Diet-1200 Cal*
50-Day Flex Diet-1500 Cal*
30-Day Quick Diet - Women*
30-Day Quick Diet for Men*
30-Day No-Cooking Diet*
30-Day Diet for Women - Metric*
30-Day Diet for Men - Metric*
25 Day Easy Diet-1200 Cal*
25 Day Easy Diet-1500 Cal*
25-Day No-Cooking Diet
10-Day Express Diet
10-Day No-Cooking Diet*
7-Day Diet for Women*
7-Day Diet for Men*
7-Day No-Cooking Diets*
90-Day Gluten-Free Diet-1200 Cal*
90-Day Gluten-Free Diet-1500 Cal*
30-Day Gluten-Free Quick Diet*
30-Day Gluten-Free No-Cooking Diet*
7-Day Diet for Women - Metric*
7-Day Diet for Men - Metric
7-Day Gluten-Free Express Diet*
7-Day Gluten-Free No-Cooking Diet*
90-Day Vegetarian Diet-1200 Cal*
90-Day Vegetarian Diet-1500 Cal*
30-Day Vegetarian Diet*
7-Day Vegetarian Diet*
Weight Loss for Women*
Weight Loss for Women - Metric
Weight Loss for Women - UK
Weight Loss for Men*
Maximum Weight Loss - 1200 Cal*
Maximum Weight Loss - 1500 Cal*

Weight Loss for Men - Metric*
Maximum Weight Loss- 1200 Cal*
Maximum Weight Loss- 1500 Cal*
Weight Control - U.S. Edition*
Weight Control - Metric. Edition
Professional Weight Control Women - U.S.
Professional Weight Control Women - Metric
Professional Weight Control Men - U.S.
Professional Weight Control Men - Metric
Weight Maintenance - U.S. Ed*
Weight Maintenance - Metric. Ed*
Weight Maintenance - UK Ed
Weight Loss for Senior Men*
Weight Loss for Senior Women*
Eat Smart - U.S. Edition*
Eat Smart - Metric Edition
30-Day Mediterranean Diet
Exercise Smart - U.S. Edition*
Exercise Smart - Metric Edition
Exercise Smart - UK Edition*
Total Fitness - U.S. Edition
Total Fitness - Metric Edition
Total Fitness - UK Edition
Total Fitness for Women-U.S. Ed*
Total Fitness for Women - Metric
Total Fitness for Women - UK Ed
Total Fitness for Men - U.S. Ed*
Total Fitness for Men- Metric Ed*
Total Fitness for Men - UK Ed
Senior Fitness - U.S. Edition*
Senior Fitness - Metric Edition*
Senior Fitness - UK Edition*
Computer Diet - U.S. Edition*
Computer Diet - Metric Ed*
Reliable Weight Loss - U.S. Ed
101 Weight Loss Tips*
101 Healthy Eating Tips*
101 Lifelong Fitness Tips*
101 Weight Maintenance Tips
101 Weight Loss Recipes
101 GF Weight Loss Recipes
101 Veg Weight Loss Recipes*
30-Day Mediterranean Diet*
90-Day Med Diet - 1200 Cal*
90-Day Med Diet - 1500 Cal*

* These titles are available as both ebooks and paperbacks. Our ebooks are sold by Amazon, Apple, Google, Barnes & Noble and Kobo, but our paperbacks are only sold by Amazon.

Disclaimer

This book offers general meal planning, nutrition and weight control information. It is not a medical manual and the author does not claim to be medically qualified. The material in this book is not intended to be a substitute for medical counseling. Everyone should have a medical checkup before beginning a weight loss program. Moreover, the physician conducting the medical exam should be made aware of and should approve the specific weight control program planned. Additionally, while the author and publisher have made every effort to ensure the accuracy of the information in this book, they make no representations or warranties regarding its accuracy or completeness. Further, neither the author nor publisher assume liability for any medical problems that might result from applying the methods in this book, or for any loss of profit, or any other commercial damages, including but not limited to special, incidental, consequential or other damages, and any such liability is hereby expressly disclaimed.

Made in the USA
Coppell, TX
10 February 2021

50014333R00114